EARTH - WATER - AIR - FIRE

ENERGIZE

SIXTY SECONDS TO BOOST
YOUR ENERGY NATURALLY

THE ART OF LIVING SERIES

a book by

JACQUES POLANCO II

Second Edition 2014

The Lahyt Company books may be purchased for educational, business, or sales promotional use. Online editions are also available for most titles. For more information, contact our corporate/institutional sales department: booksales@lahyt.com

Published by The Lahyt Company, LLC.
11566 Francis Lewis Blvd., Queens, NY 11411
publishing@lahyt.com
Lahyt.com

ISBN: 978-1499171105

Designed by The Lahyt Co.

In Loving Memory of
Shakiyla A. Patrick,
Brian R. Hemmings Jr.,

and to my parents.
Vanote S. Polanco, R.N.
Dr. Jacques M. Polanco, M.D.

ENERGIZE
Sixty Seconds To Boost Your Energy Naturally

The Art of Living

Medical Disclaimer

I Will Fill In The Blank

Can I find 60 seconds to increase my energy while waiting for _____ ?

CONTENTS

THE ART OF LIVING

Healthy Living
Why ENERGIZE?

PROLOGUE

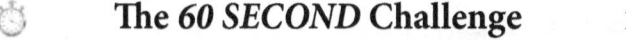

THE ART OF LIVING

HEALTHY LIVING

"Celebrating life through the elegance of natural science."

Healthy Living
NATUROPATHY

Times are changing and we need to understand that there is an Art Of Living or an art to living. Our body is the canvas and how we treat our bodies reflect in appearance, energy levels, and longevity. It takes more vibrant energy to remain happy and exhausted energy to remain sad.

I am a fanatic about finding more energy, in the next chapter you will learn why I ENERGIZE. You will usually see me walking or jogging around the neighborhood with my Jack Russell terrier, as vehicles speed pass. My trusty companion, Prince, keeps me fit and vice versa. He reminds me to enjoy the sun when we can, as well as sleep by 10PM every night by tapping me with his paw. I used to ask myself why, then I realized when I awake early I can catch more sun. Every day I jog with Prince and I arrive on one particular corner where customers are pumping premium gas in their Mercedes, that same customer crosses the street to McDonalds' drive-thru to fuel up their body. Yes the Mercedes comes with instructions "Premium-Gas Only." What instructions do we follow for our vitality? Do we care more for the look and appearance of our expensive cars? Well, our bodies crave for the same care. I rather am proactive in personal longevity than a car I can pass down. The Art Of Living is the instruction manual to maximize your daily living naturally. Behind every masterpiece is an elegant science. As with all rules and science, first know what they are and it is up us to choose which ones to break and when. Moderation. Mind Shift.

With the advances in food processing, many corresponding illnesses and conditions are also evident. Even with improvements in medical technology, you may be looking at alternative medicine as well as natural lifestyles to ensure healthy living. Like others, you may have also practiced remedies or health solutions that make use of our body's own health mechanisms and the presence of human energy. Just like acupressure, naturopathy takes advantage of the presence of vital energy within our body. In fact, naturopathy uses acupressure in treating certain conditions. Understanding of our body's processes is the foundation of Naturopathy.

In simple terms, naturopathy is the use of natural means – nutrition, exercise and botanical medicine – to heal our body. Naturopathy, according to the American Association of Naturopathic Physicians (AANP), is "a distinct system of primary health care – an art, science, philosophy and practice of diagnosis, treatment, and prevention of illness. Naturopathic medicine is distinguished by the principles upon which its practice is based. These principles are continually re-examined in the light of scientific advances. The techniques of naturopathic medicine include modern and traditional, scientific and empirical methods." Naturopathy uses different types of alternative treatment. Treatments vary from psychotherapy, reflexology and even aromatherapy.

When using reflexology, the reflexologist makes an observation of our actions first. This observation enables him to know which body part may be causing pain or limiting our ability to move. After determining the cause, he proceeds to structuring a regimen of treatment for us. Based on reflexology techniques, he begins to stimulate energy pathways within our body. By stimulating these pathways, he allows our blood to circulate smoothly. With the blood, nutrients are also delivered efficiently throughout our body. In the elderly who are not able to perform rigorous exercises, applying pressure also stimulates the nerves. It improves muscle tone and aids in flexibility or recovery for sick people.

The use of alternative treatments such as reflexology and

acupuncture or acupressure springs from the premise and the belief that our body can heal itself. Acknowledging the presence of vital energy or life force energy within our body is the first step. From there, the reflexologist or acupuncturist – as well as us – need to know where these hubs of vital energy are and how they move or flow. More importantly, we need to know how to tap into these energy sources. When we do so, we can gently massage or manipulate energy hubs.

It is not enough to know where the energy hubs are or how they function. It is also important to know what lifestyles or habits we need to be practiced and incorporated to help and maximize the presence and use of this vital energy. Aside from acupressure, acupuncture and reflexology, there are other numerous alternative treatments founded on the presence of life force energy within our body. There are bioelectromagnetic-based therapies that recognize the existence of small electromagnetic fields emitted by every cell in the human body. Through the use of magnets, electromagnetic fields that may have "relocated" or dislocated are realigned; the dislocation or relocation of such electromagnetic fields are responsible for disease.

Then there are biofield therapies. These therapies recognize the existence of energy within and around the body. Healing of our body, as well as our mind and spirit, is done by manipulating this life force energy. Manipulation takes the form of therapeutic touch or massage, qi gong (manipulation of the life force energy to improve circulation and immune function so that balance and harmony of the energy within our body is restored) or Reiki, which uses the hands to channel energy for healing.

As mentioned, our body possesses an energy. The energy in our body travels throughout it via pathways called meridians. Meridians provide a guide through which energy from organs or energy hubs flows. It is by manipulating these meridians that the body is allowed to heal. When we block the energy that is meant to flow our body may experience pain and discomfort.

In the field of esoteric science, it recognizes that the energy exists within each one of us. The activities that we choose to undertake generates energy. Therefore, the esotericist learns to channel these energies to help humanity. Ordinary people like us can, too.

Esotericism also maintains that physical ailments are only manifestations of an underlying problem. Healing is made possible through a holistic approach. By holistic approach, we are considered as a person that is not just made up of our physical body but also by our mental/emotional and spiritual self. Pain in the physical body, such as headache, may only be a symptom of being stressed.

We may be overwhelmed by our work or our responsibilities to our family that the stress we experience becomes a headache. Thus, our mental/emotional state translates to a physical condition. With a holistic approach, the stress is addressed to relieve the pain of our headache. We might be advised to get a massage or nerve manipulation. Applying strategic pressure eases out the stress and helps us relax. In addition, we will also be taught breathing techniques to enable our energy to flow smoothly. Being mindful and mastering anxiety is lifestyle changes that assist in lessening stress. They can be as simple as recommending a healthy diet and regular exercise.

When we make it a habit to consume only natural food and maintain our weight and fitness naturally through regular exercise, we become full of energy and vitality. We have a zest for life which will motivate us to pursue passions and dare us to take on challenges. We will not be afraid to make a mistake because we know that we have the vitality to do things again but in a different manner. This vitality is what drives us to perform even seemingly difficult tasks. And like every activity that generates its own energy, things can take a life of their own.

Our business may prosper because of the power possessed by our employees, giving them the impetus to go the extra mile. Employees could be motivated to give value-added service that impresses a client. The customer, through word of mouth, advertises the service that she got which translates to more business and perhaps a loyal base of customers.

You might discover that there are some items in your bucket list that are left unchecked, and you finally get a chance to assess where you have been and what you have done in your life. If you have that vitality that comes from consuming natural goods, now may be the time for you to embark on that unchecked item. You might want to go on a road trip, a fishing and trekking adventure or a cruise.

You may be an athlete or a sports enthusiast, but you cannot seem to improve your performance because you lack the power to jump higher, run faster or endure an uphill climb. The answer may lie in your current lifestyle. Instead of gulping energy drinks which contain lots of sugar or artificial sweeteners, why not try energy juices? To be able to maximize oxygen in thin air, why not learn breathing-techniques that help you conserve energy?

There are myriads of things that we can achieve and do well if we turn to the principles adhered to in naturopathic medicine. Having the energy to perform so many tasks can do well to boost our confidence and encourage us to do more. To get the energy that we need, we can turn to nature's bounty – food. The primary source of food for both humans and lower forms of animals are plants. Plants produce fruits that contain glucose that is easily transformed into energy. Vegetables contain minerals that are needed to make energy all throughout the day. Likewise, plants produce grains, root crops and beans that supply us with carbohydrates and protein to power our body's daily activities.

Naturopathy is the core of The Art of Living. So, when we consider the value of naturopathy, we can conclude that the ways to healthy living do not involve expensive treatments or sophisticated lifestyles.

All we need is to have a healthy diet, regular exercise and the intake of herbal remedies if necessary. Herbal remedies can take the form of tea or food supplements. On top of that, we can benefit from a relaxing massage, acupressure or reflexology. Furthermore, naturopathic medicine has been admitted no less than by the World Health Organization as a conventional health care system. Wouldn't you want to get a lot of major benefits without the attendant costs? Let's join the revolution of celebrating life through natural science.

WHY ENERGIZE?

Why is an artist concerned with getting ENERGIZE'd? Well throughout my life I have been slim and weak. With a super-charged metabolism, I was feeling symptoms similar to Chronic Fatigue Syndrome. My body was craving for natural fuel and improved maintenance. Even a stroll in the shopping mall was a daunting task. I was the nag who wanted to go home early from the events. You see I too use to calorie count. My Caribbean parents believed that the extra weight meant that you were healthy. I figured if I ate over 3,000 calories a day. I too can pack on pounds and increase my energy level by consuming as many calories as I could in a sitting. So I used to spend around $23 Friday evenings to bulk up by counting calories on the McDonald's menu. Boy did I love my double quarter pounders with cheese. Did I finally gain weight? I sure did! So from always driving, sitting at work, and bulking up on calories. I was a greasy and full looking gentleman with having to suck in his gut all the time. And what was even worst was when I got sick; I would lose all the body fat and my emaciated appearance was the visual proof I was sick. So I added multivitamin pills and exercise fads to my daily routine. Clearly it was time for a change, but with not enough hours in the day who has time to live against the status quo? I was tired of being tired. Then I remember something my mom said, "There has to be a natural solution." I took the stand to turn off the television programming and start listening to my body.

The adjustments were simple mind shifts. For example instead of concentrating on inhaling, concentrate on exhaling a little bit longer so that when you inhale you fill your lungs with new air. That information sure would have been handy while playing saxophone solos during my wonder years.

Although I am still slim. I am a confident slim. I no longer count calories. I walk instead of drive and stretch instead of sitting at work.

You are what you eat, so I started eating healthier. Now fatigue either means I need to take a power nap or I need to sleep for about eight hours.

So that was my past. Now let us take a new breath as we explore the elements of this book.

PROLOGUE

INTRODUCTION

As we get older and take on more responsibilities, we can start to feel like The Walking Dead. When we do not keep our life in balance and our health at the top of our priority list, it can affect our energy levels not to mention our overall health. Many of us, if not all of us, feel like there is so much to do, but so little time in this race called life. We race from one thing to another, without even experiencing the event. We might have eaten, but we most likely did not savor what we ate. We took a shower, yet we feel like water was only sprinkled on our bodies. We see ourselves in the mirror, yet we may not notice that our collars were not properly turned right-side-out.

We were supposed to go through life, enjoying every minute of it – the ups and downs. We would not be able to compare if a moment were truly joyous and ecstatic if we had not experienced pain and sadness. Sadly, we cannot enjoy it merely because we feel tired and perhaps a little bit under the weather. Fortunately, there are things we can do and food and beverages we can take to increase our energy and even enhance our performance. Such activities and nourishment can improve our quality of life.

We can ingest beverages that are energy boosting, including natural water. Water not only hydrates our body but also energizes muscles. The body also needs salt and sugar, but in moderation. Certain foods can also boost our energy; they are nutritious, as well. Modifying our diet could be all it takes to improve our performance and productivity while ensuring a remarkable quality of life. Making a decision towards a healthy diet and you'll suffer less from preventable diseases or avoid them altogether.

Regular exercise is a regimen, which may seem to expend your energy, but are energy boosting. Our Energy Case Studies will demonstrate who uses energy boosting. Stretching is also a vital component of a regular exercise, we will get into that in the coming pages. Stretching warms up the body and preps it for more physical activities. Aside from regular exercise, getting enough sleep is also a must to boost your energy. You need enough sleep to maintain our energy balance. Otherwise, sleep deprivation will reduce energy expenditure and make you feel like The Walking Dead. Other activities that may seem inconsequential are nurturing balance, reflexology, relaxation, and deep breathing.

Moreover, to help you understand and be able to apply all the energy boosting techniques that are available to you, you will come across concepts like stress, fatigue, meridians, and the four classical Greek elements and how they impact your life. There is even a discussion on how to maximize the benefits of energy boosting in just sixty seconds. More importantly, since this is a book on boosting energy, you will also learn how to evaluate and conserve energy. All these activities can be incorporated into a healthy lifestyle so that you will learn the importance of living in the present and productivity can be maximized.

This book does not list all the elements you should stay away from, but instead embraces the fundamental science behind a productive and energized life. You will also learn the seven personal side effects I experienced in the process. All I have to say is feeling energized is addictive. I'll take a long-lasting boost of energy over a short one any day. Today take the Double P.L.A.Y.Y. Approach.

"Action is the foundational key to all success." — TONY ROBBINS, American life coach, self-help author and motivational speaker

MY MOTHER A BEAUTIFUL GENIUS

"The genius of woman is the genius of humanity, the ability to love others more than one loves oneself, and love, humanity, is the supreme form of intelligence" — Dr. Ashley Montagu[1]

They say when God created us; He first created man, Adam. Eve was only created second and her sole purpose at first was to keep Adam company. Then everything changed and the world evolved. Now, women are considered vital part of the community. Their role now is more than just to keep a man company, but they possess the greatest gift any other person could have: the gift of bearing a human being inside their womb and giving birth to a child and creating a new life. To most people, women, men and children alike, motherhood is a gift that can never be replaced by any riches or jewels in this world.

How does a woman become a good mother? How does a mother rear her child to become healthy and responsible adult and citizen of our community? Know-how to becoming a good and efficient mother is not available in the market or bookshops because being a good mother is different for each and every mother. It all depends on the principles they live by, the environment they are in and the life they are living. But there is one common theme in motherhood that makes it possible for a child to become a loving, caring and responsible adult and endure any trials that life may throw at him and this is the "mother's love."

According to Dr. Ashley Montagu who had written many books that emphasizes the supreme importance of a mother's love:

> The basic plan of the mother-infant relationship, from conception to birth, and onward is that the loving behavior of the mother and child for one another confers survival and growth benefits upon each

other. In this beautiful mother-and-child interconnectedness and interaction the essential pattern is laid out for humanity to follow toward the achievement of healthy growth and development, that is, to live as if to live and love were one. (Montagu, 1996).[2]

A mother's love is the greatest weapon and tool that a mother can give to her child to make sure that her child will be able to live a healthy and good life. But aside from a mother's love, what are the other important aspects of motherhood and parenthood? A mother's love is fueled by her passion for making sure that her child is safe from harm and at the same time growing up to become responsible and loving individual. But a mother's love is best express by mentorship and by allowing the child to grow and evolve on his own.

Vanote S. Polanco, R.N. is my genius mother. As a woman, wife, mother, and registered nurse to name a few of many hats, my mother's love was expressed through her preservation of balance from maintaining homes, gardens and nutrition. She always seems to have a natural genius for blossoming plants in her garden to being a rock for the family. In my mother's elegant years, she would maintain a holistic approach to preserving her peace. She also believed that one can find solutions and remedies naturally. My mom introduced me to juicing. She loved her juicer so much she bought me the same model. Thank you mommy.

So, can we consider our mothers as geniuses? I say yes. Without them, we are nothing. How would we nurture balance? Without their sacrifices, love and support, we will never be enjoying the life that we are living now. But of course, we cannot leave out our fathers. They are the other halves that complete our identity and essence as human beings. My dad provided direction and my mom nurtured correction.

— MOTHER EARTH —

[1] Montagu, A. (1992). The natural superiority of women. New York: CollierBooks. Retrieved February 24, 2014 from http://www.thenurturingmother.com/Ashley_Montagu.html.

[2] Montagu, A. (1996). *The elephant man*. 3rd ed. Lafayette: Acadian. Retrieved February 24, 2014 from http://www.thenurturingmother.com/Ashley_Montagu.html.

60 Second Stopwatch

When I hear of a stopwatch or its uses, the first thing that probably comes to mind is an athletic event. It would most likely be in track-and-field where accuracy is essential. But to ordinary mortals like us who may not dream of beating the clock in a sporting event, the stopwatch can be a friend that helps us monitor how long we've practiced deep breathing or to gauge our heart rate. As much as it is used by coaches and trainers to gauge the performance of an athlete, stopwatches can also be a tool for us to be victorious over unhealthy habits.

I can use a stopwatch to determine my pulse rate after I exercise. Even if I do not pump iron or hit the gym, I can still burn calories or engage in beneficial physical activity for just 60 seconds. While working in Corporate America, I used to tackle the incoming calls by stretching and jogging in place. In 60 seconds, we can scale more than three flights of stairs and get your heart rate going.

Sixty seconds may be all it takes to start a healthier lifestyle. Once you start incorporating those 60 seconds into your lifestyle, the accumulation of those 60 seconds may turn into 60 minutes. Eventually, those 60 minutes can turn into 60 hours of regular exercise spread over three months. It takes little tweaks to make a significant positive change in your life. If you start healthy breathing even with just 60 seconds, you can achieve numerous benefits that improve your performance and productivity, as well as your quality of life.

Such benefits include the following:

1.   Quality of life is improved because deep breathing detoxifies and rids your body of toxins.

2.   Healthy breathing helps you relax and relieves tension

arising from emotional problems.

3.   Healthy breathing eases pain and lifts your mood.

4.   Healthy breathing strengthens and tones your muscles and aids in circulation by massaging your internal organs, including your heart.

5.   Healthy breathing boosts your energy by taking in oxygen that is circulated among the cells, thereby providing you more energy. And because more oxygen is taken in, your immune system also benefits. More oxygen likewise burns excess fat.

See what 60 seconds of exercise or healthy breathing can do? All these benefits can be regulated by a stopwatch – an invention credited to Samuel Watson in 1695; Samuel Watson was a clock and watchmaker. The invention wasn't initially called a stopwatch but a physician's pulse watch, so called because the watch was commissioned by Sir John Floyer. Floyer was a physician who needed to measure precisely the pulse rates of his patients. So the idea was Floyer's but the execution was done by Watson.

Originally, the stopwatch was made to be used as a tool in clinical practice for a physician. It can be used accurately to measure pulse and heart rates today as well as when it was invented; there is more accuracy in a digital stopwatch than in analog. More than that, a stopwatch can be used when doing exercises or training for a sporting event, even if you are just an amateur. You can monitor how long you are able to complete an action, like swimming one lap. Based on your past performance, you can train harder to beat your previous time. You can also set a time goal that limits performance of an action only within that time.

When you exercise it is helpful to check your pulse rate. Checking your pulse rate is essential because it can signal erratic conditions of the heart that might merit a visit to the doctor. A fast pulse rate even when you are resting can be a sign of heart disease or that blood is not being pumped properly by the heart. Pulse rates can be checked by feeling the area where an artery passes near the skin. Often, it is on your wrist or the neck, where the carotid artery passes.

Use your index and middle fingers when checking your pulse. You can count the times your artery bulges in one minute, or you can just count for 20 seconds and multiply it by three; counting the beats for one whole minute is more accurate.

Medical necessity help creates the stopwatch. Even today, its use is not limited to gyms, sports arenas and the playing fields but also in homes. It can be used to monitor your pulse before and after you exercise. Any anomalies with your pulse or heartbeat can prevent you from suffering conditions such as a stroke. Just a 60-second count of your pulse can warn you of possible conditions that can preclude you from enjoying a good quality of life.

And even with a very hectic schedule that would deter you from regular exercise or other enjoyable physical activities, you can still prepare your day with several 60-second physical activities like stretching and taking the stairs. Besides, they can take away the boredom of being confined in a cubicle for most of your waking hours. Those minute 60 seconds may not seem much, but they are quite significant for your health that your body will thank you through a longer and better quality of life.

Last, but not the least, the contribution of 60 seconds of healthy breathing benefits not just my lungs or other body parts involved in breathing, but optimizes the performance of other organs, as well. Moreover, your emotional life can profit from healthy breathing by relieving stress. In turn, the people around you, especially your family, friends and co-workers, feel at ease when you are around because you radiate harmony and peace. Those precious 60 seconds have a multiplier effect that goes beyond your immediate sphere.

"Am I prepared to spend all evening waiting on my car at

the mechanics? … Do you think I can find 60 seconds to increase my energy while waiting?"

"Am I prepared to binge on a season or two of your favorite show? … Do you think I can find 60 seconds to increase my energy while watching?"

"Am I prepared to spend an afternoon waiting on the line for a roller coaster ride at the park? … Do you think I can find 60 seconds to boost my energy while waiting?"

I am not constantly looking at my stopwatch, but I am mindful of finding time and rhythm to boost my energy. This book presents an understanding that all of life is complemented by nature. Anything that we need to evolve and heal can be found naturally. I feel the effect of natural stimulus within 60 seconds.

Not enough time? Not enough energy?

THE *60 SECOND*
CHALLENGE

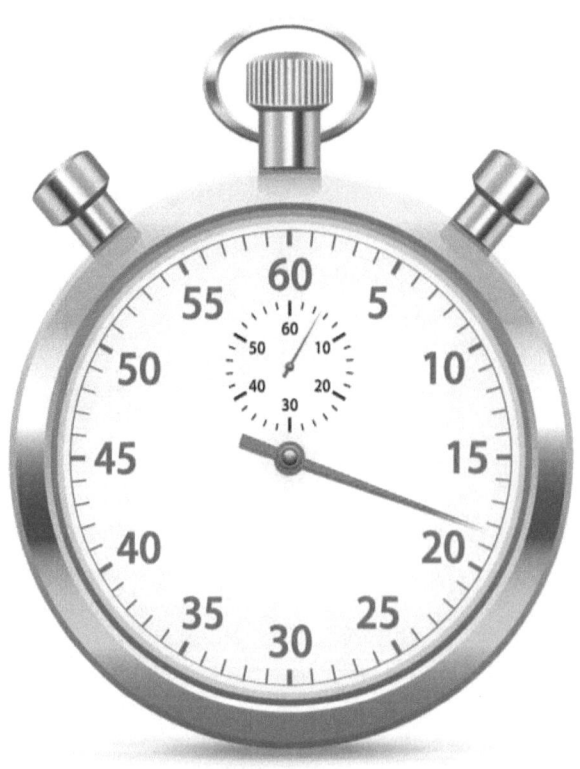

"Healing in a matter of time, but it is sometimes also a matter of opportunity." — HIPPOCRATES, Ancient Greek physician

Simple Breathe and Relax Exercise

When I am looking to peek my performance before I jog and during jogging I concentrate on my breath for endurance. The technique I use to conserve energy is I focus on exhaling longer than when I inhale; inhale through my nose. Also, do not force your lungs when you exhale. Otherwise, you would be exerting effort that contradicts your intention to conserve energy.

THE CHALLENGE

Before you go walking for 10 minutes
concentrate on your deep breathing for *60 seconds*.

Did you notice any euphoric effects?

PART I:
THE WALKING DEAD
vs. ENERGIZE

And what is a man without energy?
Nothing - nothing at all.
— MARK TWAIN

CHAPTER ONE:

FEELING LIKE THE WALKING DEAD

Ever felt like a zombie lately? That feeling you get when doing a job requires more energy than you can muster? And you feel like you are headed nowhere fast? That feeling when a simple job like folding clothes may take a whole half hour when you used to do it in just a couple of minutes? You may reason that you are tired because you have been doing a lot lately. You feel like you have overstretched yourself beyond what you routinely do or are capable of doing. Conversely, why not check if you might be lacking some nutrients? Are you eating the right kinds of food? Are you sleeping enough? I remembered when sleep was not a priority.

Perhaps, due to hectic schedules where you do not get to make homemade healthy food, you also miss out on getting the right nutrients. You may be experiencing what is scientifically defined as fatigue. It may be physical fatigue where you are unable to perform physical activities or performance of them takes a lot more energy. It may also be mental fatigue where you cannot concentrate properly or are sleepy. Mental fatigue can be caused by stress or depression, as when one suffers from bereavement or divorce or change. Change can happen when you are in a new job, new school or new neighborhood.

Physical fatigue, on the other hand, can be caused by the lack of certain nutrients, like vitamin D. Vitamin D is an energy-boosting nutrient that improves the performance of the mitochondria – the battery – of the cell. When the cells' performance is improved, the muscles are also in tip-top shape. Strong muscles facilitate snappy movements by the body.

There are many sources of vitamin D. Foremost of them is sunlight. Simple sun exposure early in the morning, when sunlight is not at its hottest and is less damaging to the skin, is ideal. You do not have to wait for your skin to bronze to get vitamin D. Otherwise, getting sunburn or exposing your skin when the sun is at its zenith might only cause you to get skin cancer.

Likewise, getting a little boost from the food you eat also combats fatigue. You can get that increase by eating energy boosting foods like peanut butter sandwich, with the bread made of whole wheat. It has to be made of whole wheat so it can be digested much more slowly than ordinary white bread. This slow digestion increases your blood glucose, which powers you up. The protein in peanut butter primarily supplies power. Any combination of protein with complex carbohydrates from whole wheat bread or crackers can be an energy-boosting snack. Similarly, starting your day with breakfast containing complex carbohydrates or high fiber, like cereal, makes sure that you stay alert the whole morning.

So as to avoid either mental or physical fatigue, you can learn to conserve your energy by:

- Controlling your breathing

- Reducing stressful activities

- Organizing your time, space and activities

- Maintaining a good posture

- Practicing relaxation, and

- Using proper equipment

Healthy breathing and relaxation shall be discussed separately and at more length in the next few pages. These simple tips can give your spirits a lift and makes it possible for you accomplish more. Conserving your energy makes you appreciate how your body works and what fuel, in the form of nutrients, can keep it going to maximum performance. Knowing the nutrients you need and their sources can help you decide on your diet.

You also have to evaluate your energy levels to gauge your physical performance. By evaluating your energy levels, you also become aware of your blood sugar and glucose levels. Having a healthy blood sugar level alerts you to the possibilities that are around you. Thus, you are assured of meeting success in your endeavors. Awareness of your energy levels also helps you organize your time with the corresponding activities. Awareness means better time management and spending quality time for yourself and your loved ones.

Most importantly, boosting energy the natural way has benefits in the short term as well as in the long term. In the short term, it improves productivity – whether you are an office worker, a homemaker or even an athletic teen. It also improves your performance because you are able to concentrate. In the long term, your ability to breathe well makes for healthy living and longevity. When you have mastered relaxing at will, your stress levels are lowered and you take in life as it comes without getting overwhelmed by its pressures.

Chapter Two:

Stress in Everyday Life

Stress is a fact of life. According to Melinda Smith, et. al. on Helpguide.com's website, stress is a normal response when you are confronted with a situation that troubles you, whether it is real or imagined.[1] When there are important and urgent things that need attention, you are bound to experience it. A bit of stress is good for you. It can enhance your "fight or flight" response and make you more adaptable to changes that happen in your life.

Managing stress is important so as not to be overcome by stressors. Start with a healthy lifestyle. Eat nutritious food, get enough sleep and exercise regularly. Avoid vices, such as alcohol, drugs, cigarettes and gambling. Take time to relax and have fun. You can also get to know how your heart responds when experiencing stress during a stress test. Stress is mimicked by subjecting the person to intense physical activity like walking or running a treadmill or using a stationary bike.

It is important that your heart functions properly because it is responsible for circulation. Circulation, through the blood, carries with it the nutrients needed by the body. Even the brain benefits from limiting the stress experienced by the body. When stress and anxiety are limited, synaptic firing in the brain is enhanced. This means that more connections are made by neurotransmitters in the brain, allowing them to communicate with each other and other body parts. The result is a more efficient body.

A more efficient body can improve productivity through time management. Better time management equates to less stress because you are able to distinguish between the important and the unnecessary tasks. Knowing what is important helps you prioritize. When you prioritize and manage your time, you are not in a hurry so you do things well. Doing things right the first time means no back jobs and less effort expended.

A more efficient body is also a product of health management. Good health management means taking advantage of stressors instead of being overwhelmed by them. Proper stress management requires that you live a healthy lifestyle, which includes a healthy diet, regular exercise and relaxation. Moreover, proper health management ensures that the nutrients you take in are distributed all over your body in areas where they are needed most. Brain function, like thought processes, memory and synchronizing body functions, is delivered more efficiently by the brain.

This takes us back to the value of boosting energy through energy boosting foods, regular exercise, good sleeping habits and relaxation, which are the same ingredients for fighting stress and managing your time and health. Once these techniques are practiced that they become a habit, you become more productive and happy. Less second-guessing your decision. Your relationships with your family and friends improve because you are able to give them quality time.

---

[1] Smith, M., Segal, R., & Segal, J. (2013, December). Stress Symptoms, Signs & Causes: Effects of Stress Overload. Retrieved February 21, 2014, from Helpguide.org: http://www.helpguide.org/mental/stress_signs.htm

CHAPTER THREE

ENERGY DRINKS VS. ENERGY JUICING

You might think that the easiest way to get an energy boost at any time of the day is to consume a whole bottle of energy drink. Not so fast. Energy drinks contain a whole lot of caffeine, sugar or other stimulants or drugs. They contain much more caffeine than in tea, chocolate beverages and soda. And since they also include an abundance of sugar, crashing down can happen after the effects of the drink wear-off – about five hours after drinking. Crashing means that your blood sugar has plummeted. A low blood sugar level can make you jittery. So the jitters can come from the sugar, not the caffeine.

Caffeine is the main ingredient in an energy drink. Caffeine is a substance that causes the release of adrenaline by the adrenal glands. Adrenaline is responsible for the energy boost when you engage in highly vigorous activities. Caffeine can be derived from coffee or guarana seeds, with the latter having more caffeine than coffee. Ginseng may also be added to energy drinks for its ability to improve overall health and stamina. Energy drinks that claim to be sugar-free have artificial sweeteners in them. Artificial sweeteners do not contain calories so they are inducements for people concerned with gaining weight or diabetics.

Added sugar in energy drinks, on the other hand, is known to contribute to obesity and diabetes. Since added sugar has no nutritional value, people who rely so much on energy drinks and do away with natural or organic foods may have poor nutrition. And if they do not brush their teeth, floss or use mouthwash, they are setting the stage for bacteria in the mouth to flourish. That can lead to tooth decay. Consuming much added sugar (and energy drinks contain a lot) also increases triglycerides in the blood stream which greatly plays a role in heart disease.

Fortunately, there is a healthy way to get an energy boost – by extracting the juice of fruits and vegetables. Everybody knows that a healthy diet comes from eating fruits and vegetables. What is more wonderful is that they can also be enjoyed in juice form. Just as it can be fascinating to be mixing alcoholic drinks for a cocktail, juicing also has an appeal because of its resulting color and taste. However, juicing does not make you feel sleepy or as a zombie. Quite the opposite. Juice from vegetables and fruits complement a healthy diet and weight.

Just because you are encouraged to drink health juices does not mean that you can disregard simple rules of cleanliness. That means cleaning your juicer once you've finished. You may use it again in a couple of hours, but that does not give you license to propagate bacteria or fungi through your juicer. By the time you mix a new batch of greens for an energy drink, it could be laced with live bad bacteria.

Instead of drinking for your health, you could end up with food poisoning. You would not want that to happen would you? Right after I juice, I rinse water-submersible parts of the juicer in warm water to quickly clean off the oxidizing fruits and vegetables.

Another thing is to limit your addition of sweet fruits so you also limit the sugar content in your juice. It is better to make it vegetable-based. So, drink up! And live it up!

Chapter Four:

Sugar, Sugar

Previously, I mentioned the negative effects of taking too much sugar as part of energy drinks: tooth decay, poor nutrition, obesity, diabetes and an increase in triglycerides. So why haven't they been banned? It is impractical that they should be banned since they add taste to food. Imagine what it would be like if what we eat were bland. Moreover, sugar aids in the preservation of jams and other fruit preserves while adding texture and color to baked items and enabling them to rise as well as adding volume to ice cream. In cooking, it neutralizes the acidity of vinegar and tomatoes.

While sugar may be deemed a necessary evil, certain types of sugar can do excessive damage. Among them is high-fructose corn syrup. It is a food additive that can be found in processed sweet snacks like

Oreo cookies, juice and energy drinks, sodas, muffins, breakfast cereals and more. Fructose in processed foods is not metabolized by the liver as fast as you take them. This further burdens the workload of the liver and thus, its recourse is to turn fructose into triglycerides. Triglycerides increase your risk of heart disease and stroke. You do not have to avoid totally some snacks to be free of a high-fructose diet.

Moderation is key. To see if you've had enough sugar on average, you can check your blood sugar levels through any of the following tests:

- fasting blood sugar

- 2-hour postprandial blood sugar

- random blood sugar

- oral glucose tolerance, or

- glycohemoglobin A1c

The first three measures your blood glucose level relative to when you have last eaten, the fourth checks how your body processes sugar and the last one measures the amount of sugar that remains in your red blood cells.

You may decide to undergo these tests if you feel symptoms of high blood sugar, called hyperglycemia, like thirst or a constant need to urinate. More telltale signs of elevated blood sugar levels include headaches, difficulty in concentrating, hunger, tiredness or blurred vision. There are also people with low blood sugar levels or hypoglycemia. Hypoglycemic people have similar symptoms with hyperglycemic ones like blurred vision and tiredness. They also experience a rapid heartbeat, nervousness and mood changes. Testing for blood sugar levels is a way to prevent the development of diabetes and change your diet accordingly.

Having diabetes may affect your quality of life and limit your food choices. There are simple decisions that can be made in 60 seconds to improve your sugar intake. For one, snack on healthful and nutritious foods. For a moderate amount of sugar, snack on salads or drink energy juices made from vegetables and flavored with fruit. Occasionally, if you cannot resist snacking on pastries or pasta, just pair it with clean water so that the sugar gets diluted. And if downing sugar-rich foods has already become a habit, just think that doing so increases your chances of getting wrinkles even at a young age.

As in everything, moderation is key. Consuming a small amount of sugar in your diet is okay. Sugar is still needed by the body to produce energy. Too much of it though, can lead to damages in the organs and can result to diseases like stroke or organ failure.

ENERGIZE – CASE STUDY #1

You might think that this book is just something to while away the time. You might think that the contents of this book are something easier said than done. You might even think that the suggestions in this book are impractical because even if you are encouraged to take the reins of your life rather than be enslaved by it, life has a way of dealing you with hard blows. Anxiety and stress are facts of life that you just have to bear. Yes. Experiencing anxiety and stress is a part of life. But it can be managed. Several energy boosting techniques that deal with overcoming anxiety and stress are suggested. And other people have benefited from applying the suggestions.

A lot of famous people practice yoga for different reasons. Madonna is one of them. She does this because it is a good cardio workout and uses the weight of her own body for resistance and strength training. As a performer/dancer, Ashtanga yoga enables her to perform dynamic movements. The model, Gisel Bundchen, also practice Anusara yoga because it keeps her in shape. And who is not familiar with Iron Man? The man behind the iron mask, Robert Downey, Jr., ascribes yoga as a support to help him perform his job.

McKernan, D. (2012, March 14). 13 Celebrities who practice yoga and why. Retrieved March 26, 2014, from theultimateyogi.com: http://www.theultimateyogi.com/13-celebrities-who-practice-yoga-and-why/

PART II:
WAYS TO TRIGGER YOUR ENERGY

"natural forces within u are the true healers of disease."
— HIPPOCRATES, Ancient Greek physician

"What lies behind us, and what lies before us are small matters compared to what lies within us."
— RALPH WALDO EMERSON, Essayist

CHAPTER FIVE:

HUMAN ENERGY, HUMAN POWER, HEALING ENERGY

So far, I have shed some light on the nutritive values of some foods and beverages. Taking the nutritious food sources while avoiding the damaging ones are advised. Additionally, healthful habits such as deep breathing have been mentioned. It is time now to venture further and explore more about how energy works within our body. Let's start with understanding concepts like Reiki. What is Reiki? Reiki comes from two Japanese words – Rei, meaning "God's Wisdom" or "Higher Power" and Ki that refers to "life force energy." Taken together, it means "spiritually guided life force energy."

Reiki is a method of stress reduction and relaxation and consequently healing. It encapsulates the power of touch and benefits the body, mind and spirit. In this respect, acupressure can be applied to let a person's Ki or life-force-energy flow. "Acupressure is an ancient healing art using the fingers to gradually press key healing points, which stimulate the body's natural self-curative abilities," this, according to acupressure.com.[1] It is recognized that a universal energy flows in each of us. However, when these energy networks are blocked, it can result to illnesses and stress. Restoring the flow takes application of acupressure coupled with a healthy diet and regular exercise.

Reflexology also utilizes the presence of human energy and that a person is composed of mind, body and soul. Reflexology is defined by the Association of Reflexologists as "a non-intrusive complementary therapy based on the theory that different points on the feet, lower leg, hands, face or ears correspond with different areas of the body." [2] Reflexologists acknowledge that the body can heal itself and reflexology is only a process of applying touch for energy to flow unhampered throughout the body.

In a way, humans are like batteries. We need fuel or charging so that we function properly. We get fuel from the food we eat. But humans are more than batteries. When rechargeable batteries have been used over and again leading to wear and tear, they cannot store any more energy no matter what you do with them. The only resort is to discard them. Not so with humans. The only time that a person cannot store energy is upon death. Before that, the body can be repaired. To repair my mind and spirit, I look to reducing stress through simple meditation.

When claiming that the body can repair itself, the fact that it is we are surrounded by energy fields. Human energy fields are created by movements or activities by the cells and tissues. Likewise, energy is needed by these cells and tissues to fuel their movements. Without it, the cells and tissues will not be able to use the fuel that it receives from the food we eat and the air we breathe.

Most people may not feel human energy fields but when a SQUID magnetometer is used, these energy fields can be objectively measured; the superconducting quantum interference device (SQUID) magnetometer is a tool that can measure subtle and minute magnetic fields. These human energy fields are referred to as biomagnetic fields. These energy fields may show changes that indicate disease. Altering these magnetic fields may, in turn, heal the body of that disease.

With greater information about the presence of energy within and around our bodies, several alternative medicines have been used to make the most of this experience. They are categorized as energy therapies whereby the touch is the primary technique used in manipulating the presence of energy within and around the body for healing. Moreover, since touch is used, it also brings a feeling of balance and harmony which enables relaxation.

In the context of esotericism where awareness of the presence of energy is somewhat hidden or 'further within', energy is connected to an organ or system. To the trained practitioner of alternative medicine that recognizes and uses energy for the body to repair itself, it is possible to locate irregularities in a particular organ or system which indicate disease. Based on this, acupressure, reflexology, Reiki or any other alternative medicine methods that work on the body's energy flow, is used to correct this irregularity and thus promote healing.

Meridians are the energy pathways upon which energy flows. Certain organs in the body correspond to these meridians. If a certain part of your body experiences pain or tension, the meridian corresponding to this body part is most likely blocked. Applying acupressure to the area can remove this blockage so that energy flows. In addition, blood circulation is improved and balance to the various parts of the body is restored.

Self healing or esoteric healing is encouraged because it capitalizes on the energy generated by the body. Body parts, organs and systems, function well and are at their peak if energy flows are not hindered.

Further, a healthy diet, regular exercise and good sleeping habits ensure that the vitality is achieved. A healthy diet supports the body by supplying nutrients and secreting hormones and enzymes. Cells receive proteins that allow them to carry out their specific function. Carbohydrates backed up by fats, supply fuel for the body to perform numerous physical activities. Regular exercise strengthens and flexes muscles for a fit body. Good sleeping habits synchronize the body's internal clock. You are able to engage in physical activities in your waking hours and allow your body to heal and revitalize itself when you sleep.

Everything that makes for a hale and hearty life is within your reach. You just have to develop healthful habits and appreciate the existence of your life force energy. Tapping into your own life force energy facilitates healing without recourse to synthetic chemicals that could have unpleasant side effects. Utilizing what nature has endowed on each of us gives us the power and choice to make decisions that provide balance and harmony. When you have developed habits that are good for you, you can harness the power and vitality that your body presents. As some people would say, "your body is your greatest weapon." Use it.

"I decided to take control of my life: I would become a warrior-scholar. I made up my mind to turn my body into a weapon... a weapon that would eventually set me free!" — Rubin "Hurricane" Carter

---

[1] Gach, M. R. (n.d.). Acupressure - the Official Website for Acupressure Points. Retrieved February 25, 2014, from Acupressure.com: http://acupressure.com/

[2] Association of Reflexologists. (n.d.). Association of Reflexologists - What is Reflexology? Retrieved February 25, 2014, from aor.org.uk: http://www.aor.org.uk/home/what-is-reflexology

Chapter Six

Acupressure & Acupuncture

There are several ways of giving healing touch. One of them is acupressure. Acupressure is "an alternative medicine technique which is based on the concept of life energy which flows through meridians in the body" as defined in Wikipedia.[1] It adds, "physical pressure is applied to trigger points with the aim of clearing blockages in these meridians. Pressure may be applied by hand, by elbow, or with various devices." Acupressure uses the same principles as with acupuncture. They differ only in the methods employed; acupuncture uses needles on the trigger points. Both are ancient healing arts although acupressure is older.

Because acupressure and acupuncture use your own life energy flow, it has self-curative abilities. It means that you or another person can be healed by the use of your or another person's hand. No drugs or large, electronic equipment shall be used for the healing process. This implies that side effects are not expected. Healing takes place based on your own life energy. Even if you are not suffering from illnesses or conditions like headaches, insomnia, constipation or tension, acupressure is a method of preventive health care. When you practice the principles guiding acupressure and acupuncture, you ensure a smooth flow of life energy throughout your body, preventing blockages that could lead to diseases and releasing tension that enables you to relax.

Acupressure and acupuncture rely on the pathways that link acupressure points to one another and their corresponding organs. These pathways are referred to as meridians. Moreover, meridians not only connect acupressure points to specific organs, they also help us gain spiritual awareness. Thus, harmony and balance between your body and your spirit is maintained. When you experience muscle tension, it can show in your posture, movements and even in your breathing. This results to poor blood circulation, weak genital functioning and conditions like constipation. Aligning the muscles through stretching, proper posture, healthy breathing and relaxation, is aided by taking advantage of the presence of acupressure points.

Both traditional Chinese healing techniques use every person's life force energy, making everyone capable of being healed physically, psychologically and spiritually. The body's life force energy can be directed to a body part that is ailing, injured, painful or stressed. When you are able to direct this life force energy, you feel a warmth or tingling sensation on that part upon which your hand is laid. After a while, when the warmth or tingling sensation ceases, transfer of life force energy has stopped.

You might seem skeptical about the presence of life force energy and how the emotions affect the organs in your body and vice versa. Remember, that you are a holistic being. So, what you feel affects the physical aspect of you. Therefore, treating yourself should also look into the emotional and psychological aspect of you. When you feel angry or hold a grudge against somebody, over time it affects your liver. Notice how you get red in the face when you are intensely angry? The redness is a manifestation of your liver fire rising. (Further on, you will be introduced to the elements that govern your internal organs. For now, they are mentioned in passing.)

As you nurture anger and other emotions, emotional imbalances are likely to take place. Emotional imbalances lead to conditions that upset the normal functioning of the organs like headaches and indigestion. Emotional imbalances are not limited to negative feelings. Feelings of joy can also create an emotional imbalance and affects the heart. Extreme joy that brings about stimulation and excitement causes positive stress. Positive stress arising from a promotion or a new romantic relationship can disturb the balance of the heart where the spirit resides. Anxiety to exhibit worthiness for the job promotion or new relationship is the result. Treating anxiety may call for acupuncture and is applied on the heart meridian. As with many things, experience emotions in moderation.

Keeping things in moderation and seeing to it that your life force energy is flowing unhindered require you to treat your body as a temple. Treating your body as a temple is as simple as having good sleeping habits, engaging in fitness activities, eating food in healthy recipes, paying attention to your nutrition, overcoming stress and staying healthy. Simple strategies for staying healthy mean knowing the area of the 12 meridians of traditional Chinese medicine. These meridians correspond to the heart, lungs, liver, spleen, large intestine, stomach, kidneys, small intestines, gall bladder, pericardium, urinary bladder, and the triple burner which corresponds to the thoracic and abdomino-pelvic area.

Awareness of these meridians and where to apply acupressure is essential. Massages like Jin Shin, A shiatsu, Shiatsu and bodywork therapies that are guided by acupressure points can bring about relaxation, healing and stress reduction. Acupressure also complements other healing methods like chiropractic care and reflexology. Manipulation of the pressure points by acupressure and acupuncture practitioners facilitates the flow of energy throughout the body; such pressure points are characterized by a cluster of exposed nerves. They can be found in front and at the back of the head, and front and back of the body and legs.

What is fascinating about pressure points is the fact that the ones manipulated for acupressure and acupuncture are the same pressure points practiced in martial arts. Martial arts uses life force energy for self-defense. As a self-defense mechanism, pressure points can be used to disable, hurt, paralyze or cause death to an opponent. In martial arts, proper knowledge of the area of pressure points, the method of applying an action to stimulate that point and its angle are necessary to deliver the desired result.

Using acupressure and acupuncture lessens pain caused by body aches and inflammation, maintains good health, keeps the body's energy in balance, enhances circulation, reduces stress and encourages healthy breathing. Furthermore, they can be used as part of a beauty regimen and better sex life. Using electro acupuncture promotes the release of particular peptides including β-endorphins and endomorphin; electro acupuncture adds an electric current between needles. Endorphins act as analgesics or painkillers as well as the instigator for the release of sex hormones. Additionally, they boost the immune system, fight stress, regulate appetite and add to a feeling of euphoria.

---

[1] Wikipedia. (2013, December 14). Acupressure. Retrieved March 3, 2014, from Wikipedia.org: http://en.wikipedia.org/wiki/Acupressure

CHAPTER SEVEN

REFLEXOLOGY — CARING FOR YOUR BODY, MIND, AND WELLBEING

Reflexology is a hands-on treatment that involves pressure on hands, feet, and ears. This form of ancient treatment is widely-known as an effective way to relax the body and alleviate stress.[1]

Although there are no substantial evidences to prove the origin of reflexology, researchers believe that its very first record was found in Egypt dating back since 2330 BC at Ankhamor's tomb. Several researchers coming from different millennium also noted that the origins of reflexology reach back to ancient India and China.[2] Even Marco Polo was said to be a medium who brought reflexology from

China to Europe when he translated a Chinese massage handbook into Italian.[3] Intrigued by the treatment, thousands of people studied how reflexology works; and even until today, this age-old treatment is still debated, studied, and applied.

Health Benefits

Though some people are skeptic on how reflexology benefits a person, several studies have been conducted on different types of illnesses and these have proven the efficacy of the treatment.

Among these medical conditions is cancer wherein researchers have piloted a study to 183 breast cancer patients. Those patients who received regular therapies showed dramatic improvements not just physically, but emotionally and psychologically, as well. Patients were also seen to have brought back their sense of wellbeing after a continuous set of treatment.[4] The National Institute of Health and the National Cancer Institute also state that reflexology is a great avenue to ease pain and anxiety to cancer patients.[5] That said, some patients do not see reflexology as a treatment but as a treat that alleviates their suffering condition.

Apart from reducing stress and anxiety, studies also show that this alternative medicine can effectively cure different types of health conditions such as diabetes, digestive problems, and asthma. Reflexology also provides the following benefits:

- Boosts energy and immune system

- Promotes deep relaxation and good sleeping habits

- Assists in repairing the body after radiotherapy,

chemotherapy, and other medications[6]

Adverse Side Effects

Although doctors and researchers have repeatedly stated that reflexology is safe, some people who have undergone the treatment claimed to feel tired and sick after the session. There are also cases wherein a patient felt discomfort from a vigorous pressure. Others also reported experiencing nausea, vomiting, and sweating. Reflexologists believe that these effects indicate that the body reacted from the therapy and that it is a positive thing. These events only happen to people who are sensitive to treatment. After a few hours, if not minutes, the body will start to feel relaxed and relieved from their health complaints.[7]

How Does Reflexology Work?

Until today, there are no intuitive evidences so that the mainstream medical experts can recognize reflexology; however, studies have been conducted, which resulted to several theories of how this ancient treatment works. Below are two of the most common theories that are being used today.

- **Zone Theory.** One of the most popular theories was the research done by Sir Henry Head and Sir Charles Sherrington who showed the neurological relationship between the organs of the body and the skin. This study revealed that the nervous system reacts to a stimulus.

Based on this theory, another experiment has been conducted that uses body mapping, known today as the Zone Theory. Here, the whole body is divided into 10 zones wherein each of these zones is said to be parallel to the hands and feet. This is where the concept that feet and hands mirror the body, and that internal organs can be mapped onto the feet and hands which reflexologists refer to as "reflex points".[8,9]

- Traditional Chinese medicine believes that energy or qi (chi) flows through the body. To keep the body healthy, the chi needs to flow freely. Once blocked, it could result to certain types of health conditions; and through the process of pressing the feet, hands, and ears on the reflex points, a person can experience relief from his bodily ailments.[10]

- **Endorphin Release Theory.** Endorphins, also known as neurotransmitters, are the body's natural painkillers. They can be found in the brain and all throughout the nervous system.[11] When the body is in the state of stress, it releases endorphins, which automatically decreases the feelings of pain that we feel – exactly how drugs like morphine does.[12] Endorphin and morphin, like drugs, are also known to be the body's natural mood and energy boosting chemical formula.

- Most people believe morphine is a pharmaceutical drug; however, recent studies show that our body makes its own natural morphine. What's more is that we are producing morphine the exact way how morphine in poppies are produced. Scientists believe that whenever a person feels as if they are in the presence of an attacker, morphine is released to as a defense mechanism to block out pain, either physically or psychologically.

- The Endorphin Release Theory is based on the concept

that the reason reflexology works are that the applied pressure on the feet and hands releases endorphins and morphine, which eventually reduces the pain and elevates the mood of the patient. It is also the same theory applied on some therapies that have similar modality to reflexology such as acupressure.[13]

Reflexology and Acupressure — May Seem to Be the Same but are Radically Different

Reflexology and acupressure are two healing arts that are thought to have similar bodywork techniques and benefits to people as both involve pressure to specific parts of the body; however, they are distinct and unique.

Similarities and Differences

Acupressure was first introduced in China 5,000 years ago — predating acupuncture of about 2,500 years. While reflexology applies pressure only on ears, hands, and feet, acupressure involves the entire body, specifically to what the Chinese medicine refers to as "acupoints." Like reflexology, acupressure is also based on the concept of life force, also known as energy or chi. According to specialists, chi travels through the pathways of the body called meridians. It is said that we have 20 meridians, but acupressure practitioners work around 14 meridians only. Along these meridians, there are 300 acupoints. Researchers and practitioners theorize that whenever the flow of chi is obstructed, certain bodily discomfort and diseases arise. To release the chi, acupoints associated with the illness must be pressed.[14]

Acupressure's Health Benefits and Drawbacks

Acupressure and reflexology also have similarities and distinctions regarding its health benefits and side issues. Acupressure is used by some medical practitioners to diagnose diseases. And, similar to reflexology, acupressure also helps prevent diseases and promotes overall health. Athletes and people who have laborious jobs also derive immediate relief from the therapy. Some reports also showed that acupressure made dramatic contributions in assisting emergencies like paralysis and heart attack. And more importantly, unlike surgical operations, it does not involve needle or knife to treat an illness as pressure is given using only bare hands.[15]

Although acupressure provides utmost benefits, some people are not fully convinced of how the therapy works – either the therapy could not stand on its own or that it is ineffective at all. The practice is also said to be not helpful for kidney diseases, cataract, and stomach aches. And if the patient is pregnant or have medical conditions like osteoporosis, fractured bone, diarrhea, and fever, going through an acupressure could have some adverse effects during or after the session; thus, informing the therapist about your health condition is essential.[16]

Though different in many ways, both therapies are used to treat ailments and bring relief to patients. And though they are not yet accepted by the mainstream health professionals, regardless of the theories and how they work, reflexology and acupressure does work and they provide several benefits to millions of people around the world.

Reflexology is a non-invasive form of treatment used together with conventional care. Since time immemorial, millions of people have proved to improve their health condition by undergoing a series of reflexology sessions. One is safe to receive this therapy – from newborn to the elderly. Reflexology is one of the safest medical procedures to cure many health problems. And, albeit discomfort claims, reflexology does not lead the patient to any serious harm compared to other general medical procedures.

---

[1] http://en.wikipedia.org/wiki/Reflexology

[2] http://www.medindia.net/alternativemedicine/Reflexology/Reflexology2.htm

[3] http://www.wisdomreflexology.com/History%20of%20Reflexology.html

[4] http://www.ncbi.nlm.nih.gov/pubmed/19906525

[5] http://www.mayoclinic.org/what-is-reflexology/expert-answers/FAQ-20058139

[6] http://www.wellness-solutions.co.uk/phdi/p1.nsf/supppages/4508?opendocument&part=5

[7] http://www.healthypages.com/community/threads/client-feels-sick-after-reflexology.23159/

[8] http://reflexcare.net/what-is-reflexology/

[9] http://www.takingcharge.csh.umn.edu/explore-healing-practices/reflexology/how-does-reflexology-work

[10] http://www.universalreflex.com/article.php/20040309175204417

[11] http://www.medicinenet.com/script/main/art.asp?articlekey=55001

[12] http://www.universalreflex.com/article.php/20040309175204417

[13] http://www.universalreflex.com/article.php/20040309175204417

[14] http://health.howstuffworks.com/wellness/natural-medicine/alternative/question654.htm

[15] http://www.webmd.com/vitamins-supplements/ingredientmono-1240-ACUPRESSURE.aspx?activeIngredientId=1240&activeIngredientName=ACUPRESSURE

[16] http://www.onlymyhealth.com/side-effects-acupressure-1331017432

PART III:
THE PLAN OF ATTACK

"If you don't have daily objectives, you qualify as a dreamer."
— ZIG ZIGLAR, *See You at the Top*

CHAPTER EIGHT:

STAGE I: EVALUATION - HOW'S YOUR DAILY ENERGY LEVEL

He, who every morning plans the transactions of the day, and follows that plan, carries a thread that will guide him through a labyrinth of the most busy life.
— VICTOR HUGO, French poet

Evaluating Energy

Measuring energy, without the use of instruments, may be made through mere observation. Notice how your wounds begin to heal a day after you get the wound? It does not take that long, but you'll only notice it after a day or two. You might also notice that you'll get only a few things done within a day. You seem to lag. Although energy levels start to decline as you age, you can boost them by engaging in activities that can be incorporated into your lifestyle – like practicing good sleeping habits and regular exercise.

Regular exercise boosts your self confidence. When you work out, you look and feel better. With regular exercise, too, your muscles are strengthened and give you a sense of accomplishment, thereby signaling that you are capable of doing things that most likely need an empowered will. Further, regular exercise enables a fresh and constant supply of oxygen and nutrients that benefit your brain and improves its function. It also releases endorphins and dopamine that help you relax and reduce stress. When you are able to accomplish so much due to the natural energy high, this turns into a cycle where you are more encouraged to embark on a new venture because you are positive that you can bring it to completion. This cycle gives you a sense of success.

This success is something that, regardless of the recognition you get from other people, boosts your confidence. It takes away your fear of failure. Even if you do make mistakes, they are only stepping stones to you, not stumbling blocks. Additionally, you learn from your mistakes and promise to do much better or approach situations differently.

Conserving Energy

Conserving energy is using less energy than the effort you exerted getting it. Consider the case of breathing that help you conserve energy. First, thought, it is vital to know how you breathe. Breathing happens when you take in air. As you take in air, your diaphragm goes down while your lungs expand as air occupies it. You then exhale, pushing air that has carbon dioxide with it, out. The diaphragm goes back to its previous position.

So, when conserving energy, the focus is to exhale longer than when you inhale; inhale through your nose. Also, do not force your lungs when you exhale. Otherwise, you would be exerting effort that contradicts your intention to conserve energy. Healthy breathing also entails using the diaphragm when taking in air. Remember that when you breathe or inhale, your diaphragm goes down. When your diaphragm goes down, it displaces the abdomen, making it expand. As a consequence, air volume can be accommodated by a larger space from the lungs down to a part of the abdominal cavity. Larger space translates to more air and more oxygen.

Finally, time your exhalation when you expend energy as lifting a load or just opening the door. When you breathe properly, you expend less energy. However, you need to practice so that healthy breathing becomes second nature. You can feel the difference when you notice that you are seldom short of breath or that strenuous activity or rigorous exercise does not exhaust you. Instead, you are invigorated. Breathing exercises will be tackled in depth in the section on deep breathing. Suffice it to say that healthy breathing is one way to conserve energy.

Chapter Nine:

Stage II: Development - Increase Your Energy and Confidence

"Love springs from the inside. It is the immortal surge of passion, excitement, energy, power, strength, prosperity, recognition, respect, desire, determination, enthusiasm, confidence, courage, and vitality, that nourishes, extends and protects. It possesses an external objective - life."
— OGWO DAVID EMENIKE, *You Are a Star*

Increasing Physical Activities

Increasing physical activities may be one of the hardest things to do in your desire to have a good quality of life. This is often the case if you equate increasing physical activities with regimented exercise and you've spent the entire day accomplishing your to-do list. Fret not. It just takes creativity to increase your physical activities while doing your work or errands. Take, for example, walking. If you have to take your dog for a walk, you are already doing it. And instead of walking the dog for just half a kilometer, make it one – even if it is just around two or three blocks. Your dog will thank you for it. More time out means more freedom and fun for your pet. It can also reduce stress on your part.

Though you may have very short durations of time to increase your physical activities, you can still do them. If you are at work and you need to go to the water station, you can take a longer route. That way, you also have a chance to stay up-to-date with any goings-on in the office rather than constantly burying your head in the sand. If you need to go the bathroom, you can do a few squats by the lavatory.

Whether you only insert physical activities into your busy schedule throughout the day or you allocate a great deal of time for it, those times will result to benefits for your overall physical, mental and emotional health. Regular exercise or physical activities can control your weight. If, occasionally, your busyness means devouring fast food, you can still counter its effect through regular exercise. Just do not make eating fast food a habit.

Physical activity also improves mental health. The influx of oxygen brought on by physical activities keeps your mind sharp and keeps depression at bay. Regular exercise also releases endorphins that give a feeling of happiness to those who just worked out.

Aerobic exercise also strengthens your muscles and improves your stamina in the long run. This is because you are trained to breathe faster and breathe deeply while your body takes advantage of the oxygen present in your blood. However, if you'd like a more rigorous and challenging workout, you might try cross-fit training. It incorporates aerobics, gymnastics and weight training. All these types of workout will make you strong, flexible and fast. And a session can last 15 minutes but your energy burst will last for hours.

If you choose to specialize in a cardio workout, you benefit from proper blood circulation. You also get to utilize your blood glucose so that it does not get transformed into triglyceride that is bad for your heart and metabolism. On the other hand, focusing on weight training or strength training results in strong muscles, weight loss and your ability to manage chronic conditions like heart disease, obesity, diabetes, back pain and arthritis. And you do not necessarily have to do it at the gym or buy equipment. You can use your own body to provide the weight or resistance. Weight training exercises include pushups, crunches and squats.

So whatever exercise regimen you choose, your body, mind and spirit are sure to help!

Nurture

When we speak of knowing, appreciating and getting energy boosting techniques, let us not forget to obtain nurturing balance. Nurture refers to nourishment. Physically, we get nourishment from the food we eat. Spiritually, we are supposed to get nourishment from our passions. Our passions are not limited to people, particularly the opposite sex. Passions may also refer to the amount of our fondness or enthusiasm for something, as our hobbies and interests. Passion fuels our zest for life. We do things, even if we are not compensated for it because it makes us find meaning and purpose in life.

Developing a passion and mastering or perfecting it requires a mentor. Through a mentor, mentees shadow or follow a mentor. More than learning a craft or art from a mentor, a learner also imbibes a mentor's social, spiritual and personal values. The relationship is founded on mutual trust and commitment. Aside from the mentor-learner relationship, parenthood also makes a nurturing balance possible. As with the general concept of parenthood, development of the learner's skills, talents and personality are of utmost importance. And the task of realizing that falls primarily on the mother.

From conception, until the mother gives birth and onwards, a mother knows instinctively about the potentials her child has. It is up to the mother to help her child achieve that. As the child develops from infancy, a genius mother provides a nurturing environment upon which the child grows and learns. Knowledge is what drives this growth and evolution – knowledge of the mother about the world and the things that shall be imparted to the child as well as the experience that the child absorbs while growing and evolving. As the child grows up, he/she also learns from the experiences he/she encounters.

For a mother, motherhood does not stop at her giving birth. Rather, it continues throughout the life of the child. As the child evolves, so has she also grow in wisdom and grace. She imparts her knowledge of the world to her child, so that the child does not have to make all the mistakes to learn. Mothers possess the grace needed to influence their children to live virtuous lives. Part of that wisdom and grace is love. The need for love and the giving of it start at infancy.

We all need love to feel accepted and to belong. It is an acknowledged need. When we grow up knowing what and how it is to be loved, it is easier to give it to other people. So a mother sees to it that she gives love as a way of nurturing her child, to grow and prosper. A mother nurtures for peace and balance. A person who has grown in love lives in harmony with fellow human beings as well as everything that is in nature.

Relaxation

Everybody needs rest to be able to recharge and be more productive in any endeavor. It also keeps your creative juices flowing. Relaxation should be part of your holistic approach to health and wellbeing. It reduces stress and increases your energy levels. Simple gestures like yawning, laughing and walking can already contribute to a good quality of life. Decorating rooms with colors that are apt for the activities likely to be done in that room also help. A bedroom, for example, will be more relaxing if it is painted in pastel colors of green, blue or pink.

Green is reminiscent of a forest or garden while blue resembles the color of a clear sky. Pink is like cotton candy that is soft and fluffy. But if you want to make an effort to concentrate on relaxation, try meditation. This activity requires the energy that doesn't require sweating out. Meditation is filtering your thoughts rather than letting them run wild. You can perform meditation in a quiet space which is accessible to you but does not invite distractions. The place can be your bedroom or your garden. You can prepare to meditate by reading up on some inspirational materials to help you zero in on the subject, thought, concept or idea when you do start meditating.

Taking things further, you can do yoga. Yoga is still meditation, but there are particular poses suggested to enhance your meditation experience. These poses mimic the states of nature – mountains, movements of the wind and seas, animals and even human stances. The area where you are to perform yoga poses should be spacious enough for you to move or stretch. Though the discipline is about the spirit, your body must also be groomed. You might want to shower or at least wash your hands and wear comfortable clothes that allow flexibility.

Meditation brings about peace of mind and reduces stress. People who practice meditation have reported achieving a healthy blood pressure, feeling less pain from headaches, ulcers and the muscles and joints, boosted immune system and increased energy levels. Likewise, it improves mood and behavior, creativity, emotional stability, happiness and heightened intuition. If meditation has become a part of your lifestyle, you become a better person and you live in harmony with everything around you, including inanimate objects. As a consequence, you feel one and only part of the universe.

Meditation, including yoga, encourages relaxation. So are deep breathing and rhythmic exercises. Rhythmic exercise is any activity that involves repetitive action like dancing, walking, cycling or jogging. Among different ethnicities, relaxation techniques vary. For the Chinese, they practice tai chi and Qigong. Helpguide.org[1] describes tai chi as "a series of slow, flowing body movements" while Qigong, according to the National Qigong Association "integrates physical postures, breathing techniques and focused attention." The Japanese, on the other hand, use Reiki (Reiki was described in the section on Human Energy, Human Power, Healing Energy). Americans relax through biofeedback (a way of using electronic devices to help you produce the relaxation response), hypnosis (the relaxation response is produced by way of "suggestion" that may be a phrase or nonverbal cue), deep breathing, guided imagery and progressive relaxation.

The Chinese have the most ancient techniques when it comes to relaxation. The Japanese developed their techniques in the last century while the Americans have developed relaxation techniques only relatively recently. The first two groups of people both rely on the existence of qi or the life force energy yet all three types use deep breathing as a way to relax. And just like information that has spread through the use of technology, meditation has also spread across the Western world, albeit with different ideas springing from its different origins. In the modern world, meditation is broadly defined as "a type of discipline... by which the practitioner attempts to get beyond the reflexive, thinking mind into a deeper, more devout, or more relaxed state." In the Western model, meditation is characterized by the "use of a defined technique, logic relaxation and a self-induced state/mode." [2]

The origins of meditation are based mainly on faith or religion such as the Baha'i Faith, Buddhism, Christianity, Hinduism, Sikhism, Daoism, Islam, Jainism, and Judaism. Meditation is a tool in which to profoundly be united with God and understand His teachings or to reach a state where one achieves enlightenment. Whichever method of meditation is practiced, one of the main goals is to relax and reduce stress. The good thing is that, by meditating and reducing stress, it boosts your confidence so that you do not turn to comfort food, which in turn helps you avoid gaining weight. So how about taking time to relax instead of binging?

---

[1] Robinson, L., Segal, R., Segal, J., & Smith, M. (2014, February). Relaxation Techniques for Stress Relief: Finding the Relaxation Exercises that Work for You. Retrieved March 6, 2014, from helpguide.org: http://www.helpguide.org/mental/ stress_relief_meditation_yoga_relaxation.htm

[2] Wikipedia. (2014, March 4). Meditation. Retrieved March 6, 2014, from wikipedia.org: http://en.wikipedia.org/wiki/Meditation#Modern_definitions_and_Western_models

Stretching

In the mornings, when you wake up, you probably stretch. You extend your limbs, including your lips for a yawn. Why do you do that? Is it out of habit? Or is there something more to just going through the motions without thinking about it? Whether you do it out of habit or not, stretching is good to start your day. It is a way of embracing your mornings and preparing for tasks ahead. Stretching is flexing your muscles especially when they had been idle for several hours when you slept.

Stretching is more advisable to be done after any rigorous exercise or activity so that the body is warm and has been prepped for increased blood circulation and nutrient supply. It could also prepare your mind for tasks ahead. Stretching is important because it loosens tight muscles that are often positioned differently from how they are supposed to be placed. If you spend so much time hunkering down on your desk or computer, the tendency of the muscles is to tighten into a hunched position. It is like your muscles have metamorphosed into barnacles clinging to a rock.

When you stretch regularly, the muscles are trained to be strong especially when there is a load involved. You do not need to carry a heavy load for your muscles to be stimulated, but it is enough that there is some resistance delivered by your own weight. Muscle flexibility is likewise trained so that the body part which you use for stretching and its corresponding muscle lengthens and loosens. In addition, when the muscle fibers are allowed to loosen, any kinks with the fibers are untangled. Scarred tissue is mended. And if you have injured your muscles or at least overworked them, you can try massaging them.

Muscles can also recover faster if you rest them or have good sleeping habits coupled with a healthy diet. Good sleeping habits are beneficial not only to the body but also to the mind as well; they improve memory and learning. Faster muscle recovery also benefits from relaxing activities as a sauna, a warm bath or even swimming. You do not need to be a bodybuilder to have strong and flexible muscles. Physical activities like doing household chores or workouts that are appropriate for your age can help you lose weight and lowers your risk for heart disease, stroke or diabetes.

Regular exercise also improves your endurance and increases your energy levels while benefitting your sex life. Because it is fun, it puts you in a good mood. After your workout, you can take the time to practice meditation or yoga further to increase your energy levels your energy levels, reduce stress and help you achieve peace of mind. Aside from yoga and meditation, practice healthy breathing to relax. Every physical activity you engage in helps promote healthy healing.

Whether you take daily strolls, take up a hobby such as dancing or gardening, physical activity is akin to having a well-oiled machine that runs smoothly.

Sleep

Sleep is often taken for granted as an important element in achieving a good quality of life. There could be several reasons why you do not get enough sleep. You might have had a social function to attend to or you might have partied until the wee hours of the morning to celebrate a milestone or an achievement. You might have taken a long nap or a nap taken too late in the day that you do not feel sleepy at all. It is also not advisable to do other things in the bedroom other than sleep or have sex.

Moreover, you could be just going through the motions of sleeping compared to having a restful and refreshing sleep. For one, you may not be comfortable with your sleep environment. Either your bedroom is too hot or too cold. Light seeps in from poor window treatment. Such brightness tells your body to wake up rather than go to sleep. If, during the day you yawn a lot, it may not be because you are sleepy. On occasions I had to unplug my refrigerator in my loft, because the rhythmic motor was interfering with my sleep. One of the drawbacks in living in an open layout.

Contrary to the belief that yawning signals that one is sleepy, yawning is a signal that the brain needs to cool down. You may think that yawning is also a manifestation of boredom, but it is not. Maybe, you have been using your brain for too long over a task. Yawning tells you to take a break. Besides, when you are done with the break, you might see things in a different perspective, helping you come up with a solution to a problem or task, which you have been working on for too long. When you yawn during a meeting and it seems that the whole world, or at least your officemates yawn with you, it could only mean that your group needs a temporary recess to let your heads cool.

When you do get a good night's sleep, you'll wake up to a person that's full of confidence and bursting with energy. More than that, a person who's had a good night's sleep lives longer. That is because the body's systems are allowed to rest and recharge while sleeping. Sleeping also affords a good memory. When you are in the process of learning something new, connections in the brain are strengthened during sleep – aiding memory. Aside from improving memory, good sleeping habits also enhance creativity.

In terms of your performance, refreshing sleep results to more stamina and less fatigue. Therefore, you can increase your productivity. Sleep also heightens your reaction time and decision making. Proper sleeping habit is most important when you are driving. When you are tired or sleepy while driving, chances of meeting an accident are heightened. If you are sleepy, you might encounter or even cause a vehicular accident. If you work in a manufacturing company and you are handling machinery, accidents or defective products might be produced.

Likewise, performance impairment is not limited to yourself as shown by the prevalence of accidents when you need sleep. You also can't perform well in the sex arena. Fatigue and low energy translate to low interest in sex. Men also have an added vulnerability – having sleep problems like sleep apnea causes a low secretion of testosterone, a hormone that is important in developing sex drive and sexual function. For women who are more conscious of the look and health of their skin, sleep deprivation can lead to sallow skin. For youngsters, sleep deprivation can lead to stunted growth because there will only be few growth hormones released.

When you do not get enough sleep, you have impaired attention and alertness and you have a problem concentrating, solving problems or even reasoning. And it is not just your brain that suffers. Sleep-deprived individuals are more at risk of developing heart disease, high blood pressure, stroke and diabetes.

If, sometimes you need sleep because of social function the previous night or you had to finish at work, you can pay up for your sleep debt by taking a power nap on the succeeding day. Taking a power nap should take only less than an hour, around 20 – 40 minutes. More than that and you might become groggy, as if you have been disturbed or awakened from a long sleep, not a nap. It could also interfere with good sleeping habits. Power naps should be characterized as being restful. A restful sleep environment should have a comfortable temperature with subdued noise and light.

Getting a power nap will empower you when you wake up. That is to say that your alertness has been restored and that you will be less likely to commit errors. Napping is also a way of getting rest. Parents with babies benefit when taking a power nap. Even if they get into sleep debt during the night, they can make installments through naps to pay off that debt.

Living

Some people often equate living with existing. But it is more than that. Living is having a meaningful and purposeful life. It also means doing things now rather than later when you forget about what you are supposed to do and what you set out to do, including realizing your plan. The things that you do, even if it seems trivial, is geared toward something that makes a difference in your or somebody's life. For example, if you are a jolly person and you like to make jokes, it can brighten someone's day. Its purpose may be to lift someone out of depression or let somebody else forget about his anxiety.

From the time you wake up, then, your morning routine should set the tone for living the rest of the day. In the morning, commit yourself to living a day with purpose. A sign that you are living the day with design is the number of accomplishments you have for the day. When you make a to-do list, see how many of those on the list are accomplished. This does not mean, of course, that you drive yourself as a slave. To accomplish much for a day, take time to go on a break. Having a break recharges and refreshes you for the next task ahead, thereby letting you do something in less time.

Limit or avoid distractions altogether so you can concentrate on a given task. Regular exercise and good sleeping habits also give you more energy so you can achieve more. You can also concentrate more on your current task if you do not worry or think about the next one. All your energies are solely devoted to the task at hand.

Yes, it is okay to learn from the past and prepare for the future but regretting past actions will only lead you into depression. Depression is a state where you are not confident of who you are and your capabilities. It paralyzes you from doing anything that capitalizes on your gifts and talents. It makes you think you do not qualify. You will think about what you should have done instead of using the present to correct any mistakes you may have made in the past.

If you worry about the future, you put yourself in a state of stress. Anxiety is when you fear that you will fail in any endeavor that you want to embark on. It steals your motivation. You end up falling short of your potential. In the twilight of your years, when you look back, you realize you could have done a lot and have wasted your time. You may not even remember what took up your time.

However, you do not have to stay depressed or anxious. Never forget that you have family and friends that you can count on for support and encouragement. Maintain a good outlook in life and make sure you get a healthy diet, regular exercise and enough sleep. If you feel stressed and overwhelmed by the responsibilities and problems that come your way, take time to relax even if it is just taking a walk, a nap or a hot bath.

Chapter Ten:

Stage III: Execution - Maintaining your Confidence (Energy for Life)

Confidence is contagious. So is lack of confidence.

— VINCE LOMBARDI, American football player, coach, and executive

THE ART OF LIVING IN THE MOMENT

Why Today is Important

Mindfulness, not multitasking, is an art to meet your goals and become a happier person. Multitasking may seem to be productive, but it is not, it the act of multiple distractions. There is no problem to put every bit of effort in your body to your goals, but if you are sacrificing "living" for the pursuit of a better future, then your present life is considered unhealthy. What does living mean? It means, enjoying life responsibly. It means enjoying today – what you have and what you do right now. It means being in the state of happiness because what you do today, what you believe in, completes you.

Why Today is Essential

Today is here and ready to take action. Yesterday is gone and tomorrow might not come.[1] If you have a chance today, grab it. It might not come back again so you better pay attention to it. Of course, your vision for the future is important, but the foundation of that future is today. What you do today, what is important to you today, what your thoughts and actions are today, mirrors your future.

Your fate is in your own hands. Your actions and your words will reflect your future. Just like if you study medicine, there is a 90% probability that you will become a doctor. If you like putting drugs into your system, then you will suffer the ill effects of drug addiction in the future. If you surround yourself with tech geeks, so you will soon be creating your very own software application.

If you spend your day stressed and full of negativities, you will create a life with similar scenarios. But if you spend it mindfully, with a grateful heart about what today has in store for you, it will accumulate into a happy and gratifying life.[2]

Is Multitasking Efficient?

In the name of efficiency, people tend to multitask; however, it is the opposite thing that always happen when we juggle schedules at a time. Research even shows that the result of multitasking is utterly inefficient. Not only do you produce unsatisfactory service to your boss, your spouse, and your family, you also put harm to your health. Multitasking divides your attention to small percentages for each task.[3] (MacMillan, n.d.)And because you are not "in the zone," you are not producing best results; introducing errors into your activities. Each specific job requires a specific mindset. It demands you as a whole. It demands you to stay there.

Multitasking kills happiness. You start missing out on your life. Checking your emails on the phone while you walk to your office and chow your snack could lead to, as researchers call it, "inattentional blindness." You start overlooking the obvious things that are in front of you. Because your brain can only do so much, other things that are not registered on your to-do lists are often left unseen.

How to become productive by being mindful

Changing a bad habit is indeed hard, but if you will not try to fix it (while you still can), you will live the rest of your life with "if onlies and what ifs". Here are expert guidelines on how to become more productive by being mindful.

1. **Introspect**.

   - This should be your first step to your life-changing journey. Introspection is your best chance to assess yourself. It is the perfect time to determine what went wrong, to mind yourself, and to stop blaming the external elements why you are not happy with the way you manage your time.

   - Schedule a long walk by the seashore or jog before sunrise. You can even enroll to a meditation class to de-stress. Take advantage of the moment that no one, even your family or friends, will come to your room to have a chitchat. Find a quiet spot – a place where you can just be yourself, where you can breathe…a place where there is no pressure. Then start reminiscing your activities from the past when you start being unproductive. Use these past thoughts as your stepping stones to correct your mistakes.⁴

   - Your past should not act as a stumbling block to moving forward. Don't dwell on your failures negatively. Get over it and move on.

2. **Become an early riser**.

   - Ask successful people in the world today on how they achieve their goals and they will tell you one thing – wake up early. High achievers and productive people have morning routines. And what do they do before 8 a.m., you may ask? Modern CEOs usually start their daily work before sunrise (as early as 4:30 a.m.), and they accomplish several tasks by 9 a.m.

- Irwin Simon, CEO of Hain Celestial Group wakes up at 5 a.m., and before 9 a.m., he has done many things such as going through mails, walking the dog, having a breakfast meeting, and checking operations online in Asia and Europe. You may think that he is multitasking, but he is not. He does all of these things separately. He is not in a rush. He is not juggling activities. He is mindful. And definitely, he loves his work and is enjoying his life.[5]

- Common things successful people do as soon as they get up from bed involves their health and tiny specks of their work. Being productive can only be achieved if your body and mind is healthy.[6] o out and exercise. Feel the air and enjoy sun exposure. Breathe. Energize. Then after sweating out, feed your mind by spending some quiet time through relaxation. When your body and mind are prepared for the day's activity, start mapping out your daily schedule before heading to the office.

- Studies show that early risers perform better. They tend to be more successful and optimistic in life. Morning sets your mood for the whole day. If you do not start your morning right, feeling lazy and unproductive, you are more likely to carry the mood all throughout the day.

3. **60-second meditation.**

- To change yourself to become mindful can be daunting especially if you have been living with a hamster wheel in your head for years. However, there is a quick exercise to help you start the journey – the 60-second meditation. This exercise will help you condition your mind to whatever is happening in the moment. It will set your power of attention. It will help you listen without judgment, accept things as they are in the moment, and act wisely to an event. In this 60-second mind exercise, you practice being in the present. Just quiet down your mind, breathe, and be grateful.[7]

4. **Do less.**

   - Ever had those piles of daily to do lists that you were unable to get accomplished? There was a poster on the Internet about an overloaded washing tub symbolizing multitaskers. The poster says that if the machine is loaded, it cannot wash clothes properly, drying takes longer, and may cause the machine to break down. This is what will happen to you when you multitask and say yes to unimportant commitments.[8]

   - The solution to this problem is obvious and simple. Do not overload. Do not over commit. Learn how to say no. Simplify things. Do your tasks separately – slowly and deliberately. So when you are walking, just walk. When you are listening, just listen. And when you are working, just put every bit of your energy, time, and intelligence into work. Once you do these, your mind will be peaceful and focused.

It is saddening. Every second of those wasted time while you multitask could have turned out to be beautiful. So exist in the moment. Fall in love with your today. Give your all, your very best. Treat today as if it is your last. No reservations. No regrets. No boundaries. Try it and you will see how this simple trick can create a positive and productive change in your life.

---

[1] http://www.heartspoken.com/3577/why-today-is-so-important/

[2] http://www.heartspoken.com/3577/why-today-is-so-important/

[3] http://www.health.com/health/gallery/0,,20707868_2,00.html

[4] http://elev8.com/178882/why-today-is-so-important-to-your-life/

[5] http://www.businessinsider.com/successful-early-risers-2012-1?op=1

[6] http://www.forbes.com/sites/jennifercohen/2013/10/02/5-things-super-successful-people-do-before-8-am/

[7] http://www.activelynorthwest.com/inspiration/living-lifewise-mindful-60-seconds/

[8] http://inspirationfeed.com/articles/self-development/5-procrastination-excuses-you-probably-use-and-how-to-crush-them/

THE *60 SECOND*
CHALLENGE

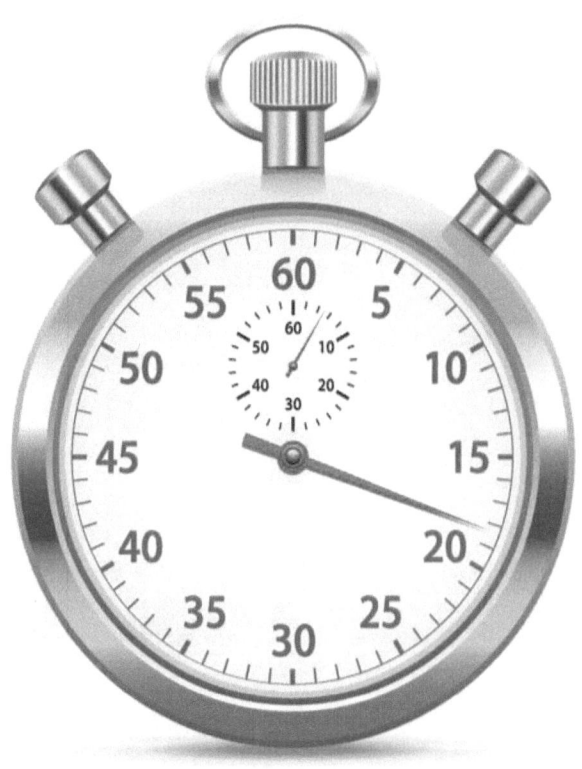

4 STEP CHALLENGE
STEP - RELAX - BREATHE & *GO*

STEP - Take the first step to start your mornings. Stand close to your bed and stretch to the ceiling.

RELAX - Relax and take a personal moment.

BREATHE - Breathe in after a long exhale inhale with a deep breath. Repeat to embrace the sensation for 60 seconds.

GO - Go ahead and start your productive day.

Join the conversation on **www.morningmats.com**

PART IV:
BACK TO BASIC ELEMENTS

Chapter Eleven

4 Classical Elements

If we look at the things around us, they come in several states: solid, liquid, gas and plasma. In ancient times, trying to understand the world around us meant classifying objects into such states. So much so that the different disciplines we have today are based on the composition of matter in these states. It has been observed and proven that indeed, all objects or matter in this world is composed of earth, water, air and fire – elements that correspond to solid, liquid, gas and plasma respectively. We should be mindful of the elements to know more about them and let us know the roles they play in our everyday life. Knowing more about them helps us use them for the sustenance of life.

EARTH

Let us start with earth. Earth is where we live and on which we build our houses. It also provides the food sources of plants and animals, which in turn, provide our basic needs such as food, clothing and shelter. It also possesses the gravity that stabilizes everything on earth. In Japanese philosophy, the earth is a symbol of strength. Within the body, it corresponds to the bones, muscles and tissues, which give form and structure to the body.

From the earth, we also get different resources, like fossil fuels, gems and other precious metals. Fossil fuels are usually made of organic matter while gems and other precious metals are just rocks, yet they command very high prices. What gives fossil fuels its status is its ability to give energy while precious metals are so dear because of their properties and rarity; most precious metals are non-corrosive and non-reactive.

WATER

Water has been equated with life. In the body, it is the transport system that carries nutrients to various parts of the body. Water is also equated with the power of flow. Additionally, it hydrates the body and makes skin supple. It is recommended to drink at least eight glasses of water, daily to keep you hydrated. Even the food that we eat, such as fruits and vegetables, contain water. Their water content allows us to juice them so that we get their benefits – vitamins and minerals – through fruit and vegetable juices.

And speaking of content, the brain is 80% water and the earth is covered with around 71% water. The irony is, potable water is hard to come by in some areas, while statistics points to the vast number of water that is around us.

AIR

Remember Pocahontas and the song, "Colors of the Wind?" It talks about the life that flows within each object on earth, whether animate – animals and birds – or inanimate, like rocks and rain. The song refers to the environment that can be found all around us. In the same way, air can also be found around us, though it is unseen. Breathing or tasting the air, as in the wind, is like embracing life's energy. Deep breathing is allowing life's energy to calm you down and help you regain your balance. You can practice deep breathing by inhaling as much as you exhale.

If you inhale for four seconds, you also exhale for an equal duration of four seconds through your nose. Another technique is diaphragmatic breathing that was explained earlier. You can also try alternating nostrils; inhale through your left nostril and exhale through your right. You can close off one nostril by pressing on it with your finger. If you want to better your performance, you can control your breathing. You can do so with diaphragmatic breathing that allows you to take in more oxygen. More oxygen, thus, travels through your bloodstream and into the body parts that need it most – like your legs when you are a runner – and of course, to your heart that pumps the blood in the first place.

When you are a mountaineer, breathing can be a challenge. Every time you inhale, there is less oxygen that goes into your lungs because the air at high altitudes is thin. So, to compensate for a little oxygen every time you inhale, you have to breathe faster and more deeply. In this way, more oxygen is taken into your body. In addition, rivers of air high above the mountains can have wind speeds faster than a hurricane. It is the same river of air that helps planes reach their destinations faster by helping propel the planes.

FIRE

The fourth element, which is often overlooked, is fire. Fire is important because it cooks our food and provides heat. When it goes out of hand, as a bush fire or burning building, it becomes dangerous. Therefore, you can say that fire can be a weapon to burn or a tool for cooking or providing heat. In person, it symbolizes your passion, energy, will and courage. Since the fire is dependent on oxygen, fuel and heat, so is a person's will dependent on his/her conscience, desire and experience. Based on them, he/she either wills to do something or omit doing anything altogether.

Physically, we get fire that powers our metabolic process from the sun. A particular metabolic process that transforms a cholesterol-like precursor into vitamin D occurs when you are exposed to the sun. Since vitamin D is responsible for the absorption of calcium for the growth of bones, deficiency in the hormone can lead to rickets in children and osteomalacia in adults. Both conditions are characterized by softening of the bones. The presence of vitamin D that supports calcium absorption in bones makes growth and development possible. It also reduces the risk of multiple sclerosis or developing heart disease.

Too much sun exposure, though, can lead to sunburn or accelerated skin aging. So it is wise to put some sunscreen on or to sunbathe only early in the morning or late in the afternoon. The warmth of the sun also provides energy to plants. It allows them to convert solar energy to simple sugars that the plants need to grow. People or other animals then consume the nutrients present in the plants. In this case, the fire of the sun is used as a tool for generating power. It is a good thing that the sun is far away from the earth that its energy is useful. Otherwise, it becomes dangerous especially because the sun is 15 million degrees Celsius hot at its core.

Now that we have discussed the four classical elements, it should be noted that all four don't exist independently of each other. The earth needs nourishment from water and energy from the fire to produce the resources that we use. Air helps sustain the life that is on earth. In short, everything, including us is part of the circle of life. These elements are not also made present haphazardly. They have to be in balance so as to allow life to thrive.

The four elements have been the foundation for modern disciplines like science and medicine. They have also been the basis for each basic unit of matter. Further, a combination of the elements resulted to a unified whole by attraction or repulsion. In Japanese philosophy, the elements relate to the different aspects of swordsmanship where the technique in handling the sword is associated with nature. As previously mentioned, the earth is a symbol of strength and corresponds to one's resistance to change. It manifests in a person's stubbornness. On the other hand, water speaks of fluidity and adaptability to change, as shown by plants that grow toward the sun.

Air or wind as commonly referred to in Japanese philosophy speaks of growth and expansion. An example of this would be the mind that grows and expands as a person develops into maturity. Fire refers to movement and energy, which is manifested in a person's passion and drive. A fifth element in Japanese philosophy is Ku or void. It represents something that is not part of everyday experience, as the ability to think and be creative. It refers to the spirit or thought and manifests itself in one's inventiveness.

Meanwhile, Western culture associates the four elements with astrological charts and horoscopes. The zodiac signs are ruled by characteristics of the four elements. People can either be extroverts or introverts, based on their zodiac signs. However way you look at the elements, whether through a Greek, Japanese, or Western perspective, it cannot be denied that they contribute much to your overall health. The earth produces the plants that you consume to provide you with the proper nutrition for a healthy body. Even the meat that you eat roam patches of earth.

Likewise, water facilitates the flow of the food that you ingest – from your mouth, through your throat and down your stomach and intestines. Water also lets you achieve fitness by providing recreational facilities where you can swim, dive, fish, snorkel, and play other water sports. Air, for its part, affords the freedom to breathe anytime you want and enables you to relax through deep breathing. Fire complements what the other elements give. It cooks your food and heats your milk so you can have a good night's sleep.

Another element that has been mentioned by the Greek philosopher, Aristotle, was aether. Aether was believed to be that void or vastness beyond the terrestrial sphere and was responsible for the circular movements of heavenly bodies. Studies by medieval alchemists called aether, quintessence. For them, since quintessence was considered pure and heavenly, it was believed to be an elixir. Aether's existence was also used to explain the behavior of light and gravity.

Chapter Twelve:

Foods from Earth that Boost Your Energy

"Let food be thy medicine and medicine be thy food." You might be familiar with this quote by Hippocrates. Hippocrates was a Greek physician and probably knows whereof he speaks. It is no wonder then, why the Greek or Mediterranean diet is commendable for those who'd like a long and enviable quality of life. Food is treated as a medicine, in that, people consume foods that have health benefits which prevents illnesses and thus, there's no need for medicine. The second part of the quote, "medicine be thy food," does not mean that popping pills regularly will prevent diseases. It essentially means the same thing: eat healthful foods so you do not have to take medicine.

Greek food is based on foods that grow – foods that come from the earth – one of Greek philosophy's classical element. And most of these foods also give energy. You can start your day with polenta. It has complex carbohydrates that are broken down slowly so that you have the energy while maintaining a healthy blood sugar level. You can course it down with a cup of coffee or green tea. To give you more energy halfway through the day, have crab-based meal for lunch. The proteins that the crab provides also regulate the release of protein-like insulin that helps you keep a healthy blood sugar level.

Pair your crab recipe with brown rice and this time you can just wash it down with water. Water has no sugar, no carbohydrates and no calories but is a healthy elixir which you can pair with any meal. An afternoon snack of whole wheat bread with farmer's cheese can boost your energy when the day is not quite done and your work is even less so. Pressed for time? Well, munching on apricots can also give you a burst of energy even while you are still busy with work. Finger foods, like almonds, can also be kept in a jar on your desk to give you a boost anytime you need it – even if it is far from snack time.

There doesn't seem to be a limited choice when it comes to eating healthful foods. Even people whose diets are restricted because of certain conditions can eat a lot of the foods that they like. It is just a matter of modifying your lifestyle so that you do not feel deprived of eating your favorite foods. Take the case of a person who has celiac disease. Celiac disease is a form of autoimmune disorder whereby eating foods with gluten, such as bread, cakes, and pasta can lead to an inflamed small intestine and may further cause complications. Gluten is a protein that is found in wheat, rye, or barley. Fortunately, there are already breads and other foods which are labeled gluten-free. Otherwise, stick to safe choices like eggs, unprocessed nuts or fruits and vegetables.

Speaking of fruits and vegetables, there are many benefits you can derive from them. Apples are good sources of vitamin C. Vitamin C is an antioxidant that discourages premature aging and the formation of free radicals that lead to cancer. Bananas support heart health and help keep a healthy blood pressure since it has lots of potassium. Carrots are good for the eyes because it is rich in vitamin A while celery is rich in vitamin K that is responsible for blood clotting. Celery also lowers blood pressure and prevents cancer. Ginger, although not a vegetable but a root, alleviates muscle pain due to exercise, inhibits inflammation of the colon and relieves nausea caused by chemotherapy.

Aside from the sweet taste of grapes, they are good fighters of heart disease and cancer due to their flavonoid and antioxidant content. Another fruit that fights heart disease and decreases the risk of stroke is kiwi. In addition, its vitamin C content makes it good food for the skin. Meanwhile, tomatoes are famous for the antioxidant lycopene and their lutein content which is beneficial to the eyes. Watermelons, including the honeydew variety, are rich in vitamins A and C. It relieves muscle pain and reduces the risk of developing cardiovascular disease. Pineapple and mango also have vitamin C and antioxidants to prevent diseases of the eyes like macular degeneration or cataract.

Pears are a good choice in reducing bad cholesterol while papayas contain folate that slows memory decline. Consuming cucumbers are good for those who are trying to lose weight. While gourd – whether bitter, bottle or some other variety – are helpful in maintaining a healthy blood sugar due to their insulin-like peptides. In general, fruits contain much water that hydrate the body and make the hair and skin healthy. Vegetables contain fiber that aids in digestion as well as containing lots of nutrients that lower the risk of heart disease, cancer, high blood pressure and high blood sugar.

Looking for healthy recipes? Try combining fruits and vegetables as you juice. An apple and watermelon juice combination can double the punch of a beverage that is good for lowering the risk of cancer and heart disease while an apple, pear and pineapple combination have an additional benefit of reducing bad cholesterol. Cucumber combined with parsley and celery flavored with ginger lowers blood pressure without putting on weight. Celery, spinach and tomato seasoned with dill controls blood pressure and help the eyes.

Since fruits and vegetables are not enough to get the proper nutrition, healthy recipes using monounsaturated or polyunsaturated fats are needed. Monounsaturated and polyunsaturated fats are good for the heart and your cholesterol level. Scrambled, sunny side up eggs or omelets, and perhaps sautéed vegetables may use olive, canola, soybean or corn oils. Healthy oils from peanut butter, avocados, nuts, fatty fish such as tuna, sardines, trout or mackerel can be ingested to promote a healthy diet.

Meals

Eating meals is as important as breathing. You need food to sustain you, especially if you are highly active. Highly active athletes, sports enthusiast and energized public figures modify their diets so that they get enough nutrients to fuel their performance. Eating wisely addresses your nutritional needs and keeps your body in tip top shape. It also staves away illness. For endurance, the pattern of eating changes. More solid food is necessary than drinking food – so protein shakes are not an option. The main source of hydration is water, helping food digestion, maintaining coolness, transports nutrients and acts as lubrication. Athletes stock up on carbohydrates when preparing for a sports event and shift to a protein-rich diet during the event.

For people who'd like to follow the diet and workout of bodybuilders, they have to eat a lot (six meals per day) but they must follow a portioning of 30:50:20 which mean that their meals must be 30% protein, 50% carbohydrates and 20% fat. Their diet intake should total 2,900 calories daily. Protein and fat based on this calorie intake can come mainly from grilled beef sirloin while carbohydrates can come from cooked brown rice. They also exercise all their muscle groups and lift different loads for variation and strength.[1]

Runners have a slightly different diet. Carbohydrates should be about 60%, protein 15%, and fats 25%. Running needs many fuels, depending on how long you intend to run for practice daily. A mile requires about 100 calories. More than muscle, fuel is needed. That is why carbohydrates constitute the greatest percentage of fuel supply rather than protein or fats. Both fats and protein can be used as fuel but can take more time to convert to fuel. Carbohydrates can be burned as fuel faster. Water intake should also be increased right before the race to keep one hydrated.[2]

For athletes, replacing meals with protein shakes may be beneficial if they are preparing for a sports event. They need the high concentrations of protein to build muscle, but consuming protein shakes for all meals throughout the day deprives them of other nutrients. Everyone, including athletes, must take in the basic food groups – carbohydrates, fats and protein – for all the organs and systems in the body to function properly. Taking in protein shakes alone will supply you with protein, water and some amount of carbohydrates and fat that are not enough to answer your daily nutritional requirements.

If you are not active, drinking protein shakes will have no effect on your muscle growth since you are not using them in the first place. You have to be active for muscles to grow and benefit from protein shakes. The same goes for replacing meals with protein shakes for weight loss. You can lose weight but make sure not to replace all meals with shakes so you do not deprive yourself of needed nutrients.Our goal is to maintain a balanced meal that includes vegetables, fruits, grains, milk, a bit of healthy oils and protein-rich foods like lean meats, eggs, fish, poultry and nuts.

Nuts and fresh fruits along with lemon flavored water (the natural kind) and whole grain bread are great natural foods that enhance your energy level. They are also good for Olympic athletes who train for endurance. Clearly, performance is improved by the combination of the four classical elements in Greek philosophy. Athletes consume food that is provided by the earth and are hydrated by ounces of water, even naturally flavored ones. Nourishing our bodies is as nourishing the earth. In turn, the body as well as the earth becomes strong. It is also implied that they have to breathe properly to maximize their oxygen intake every time they inhale. Fire, in the form of energy, is what fuels them to achieve.

---

[1] Beardsley, C., & Frank, K. (2013, January 4). How do Bodybuilders really eat and train? Retrieved March 14, 2014, from articles.elitefts.com: http://articles.elitefts.com/training-articles/how-do-bodybuilders-really-eat-and-train/

[2] Dove, L. L. (2010, July 14). What should distance runners eat every day? Retrieved March 14, 2014, from HowStuffWorks.com: http://adventure.howstuffworks.com/outdoor-activities/running/health/distance-runners-eat-every-day.htm

CHAPTER THIRTEEN:

WATER OF LIFE

As mentioned previously, water is the main source of hydration for the body because of its various roles. However, it is not just the body that needs water. Water is vital for all existence because it provides a place for marine animals to live, it irrigates fields that feed people, it nourishes vegetation that clothes people and provides shelter. More than that, it serves as thoroughfares for the transport of goods as well as people and is used in industries that provide energy and products. Water is also used as a cleaning agent, solvent and for recreational purposes like fishing, boating, swimming, or other water sports.

Water is necessary for the transport of fuel throughout our bodies. People would also be prone to choking. Also, imagine if there was no way to cool the body as manifested when one sweats. You would probably self-combust if your body's temperature is not regulated and you retain body heat. Likewise, if there were no oceans, streams, lakes and rivers, there would be no marine animals which add to the food chain. There would also be fewer sources of healthy fats from fish and other nutrients from shellfish. A lack of water would also mean a lack of food since there will be no plants that would thrive.

People would be living in caves. Even then, since caves are carved out by flowing water, people would have nothing to protect themselves. The iron ores and other materials which are yielded by the earth to build houses need to be processed to be useful. And processing requires water. That is why, if there is no water, there is no life. Those are the physical attributes and contributions of water.

In Greek philosophy, water represents adaptability – the ability to adapt to change. Like water, the flexibility to adapt to change is commendable. When you are able to adapt to change, you adjust to what life offers you. You take advantage of what is in front of you. You are realistic about what is available and you work with it. Being proactive leads to less frustration and ultimately, success. Moreover, you learn from the experience. You may encounter setbacks, but those setbacks allow you to take a different approach and get to know what works and what doesn't.

You get creative and the situation encourages you to think out of the box. Your ability to solve problems widens because your own expectations do not limit you. When you discover new things because of the experience, you get excited and your energy is boosted without taking anything. Just like water that has no additives or preservatives. It only contains two hydrogen atoms and oxygen. It is pure and simple, yet very powerful. In recognition of its power, we should also take in enough of it.

It has always been touted that we should get at least eight glasses of water a day. That is a basic requirement. But if you are an active person and you sweat a lot you might need more than that. Drink water during and after a vigorous physical activity. If you live in a place that is hot, you also need to drink lots of fluids because you may perspire a lot even if you do not perform any rigorous physical activity. If you discharge water a lot through your urine or feces, you would also need to replenish the water in your body to keep you from getting dehydrated.

Breathing also discharges water in the form of water vapor. Sometimes, when you have a fever or diarrhea and vomiting, replenish the lost fluids immediately before your condition gets worse or before you develop complications. What you should keep in mind is to drink when you feel thirsty and eat when you feel hungry. Unless when you have a medical condition, such as kidney disease, your water intake might be limited. Kidney disease prevents you from processing your food and liquid intake properly so that they tend to build up in your body and result to swelling in your calves and ankles.

However, drinking too much water is not also good. You'll know that you have drunk too much of it if you pee frequently, even when you are already in bed and your pee looks as clear as the water you drank. Drinking too much water may upset the balance of water and salt within a cell, leading to water intoxication where the cells break and you experience headaches, disorientation or vomiting. Too much water intake may also lead to cold hands or feet and insomnia.

Chapter Fourteen:

Deep Breathing

Throughout this book, you have been encouraged to take deep breaths to calm you down and help you relax. Now that you know a bit more about the benefits of deep breathing, you probably can't wait to start. When you do start, remember that deep breathing requires the proper form so that you can optimize the action of your diaphragm. More than that, you do no constrict or congest the flow of oxygen through your trachea, into the lungs and eventually, to other parts of your body. It is important, then, that you make the most out of the air you take in.

Air is vital to your existence, much more than water, because, without it, you will live only for a few minutes. Other functions in and of the body depend on it. If there is no oxygen in the body, body processes will collapse. Your brain, which needs plenty of oxygen, may not be able to coordinate your bodily functions. You get into accidents like colliding with furniture. When you are in a hurry for an appointment, you bruise your hip hitting a table because you could not correctly estimate the distance between the table and your hip. Lacking enough oxygen through deep breathing could get you confused and disoriented. You will not have the required power to engage in very simple tasks like walking or intelligible talking because not enough oxygen is burned to supply you with power.

You cannot come up with solutions or ideas because your brain lacks the needed fuel to work properly. You become sluggish and you accomplish fewer tasks, if at all. In short, you and your body cannot function well for lack of air. Plants that are sources of food for both humans and lower forms of animals die because they need air to process sunlight and water for photosynthesis. In order for the plants to grow photosynthesis needs to occur. Animals, including mankind, will also die. Essentially, you need to practice deep breathing to benefit what a free commodity can give you.

Even in just 60 seconds, you can have several repetitions of deep breathing exercises. What's more, your stomach muscles are massaged so that it can take in a variety of food without getting constipated. Deep breathing benefits different systems in the body only due to more oxygen intake. Some of them are:

• **Smoother flow of lymphatic fluid** – The lymphatic system involves the transport of tissue fluids from the intercellular spaces toward different tissues of the body. An abundant supply of oxygen through deep breathing increases the fluidity of this transport. Other nutrients are also distributed evenly throughout the body. An effective immune system is also built up and speeds up recovery from illness.

• **Cleaner body** – Perhaps unknown to many, breathing – particularly exhaling – is also a way of detoxifying. In the section on Water is Life, I noted that water, specifically its used part, water vapor, is exhaled. Since some of the discharges, wastes or excess, finds its way out of the body through exhalation, other organs responsible for excreting wastes is spared from added work.

• **Increased brainpower** – Taking in much oxygen through deep breathing means that more oxygen goes to the brain and fuels mental processes. The result: better concentration, well thought out decisions, and higher productivity and learning.

• **Better functioning of the respiratory system** – Since the diaphragm is used to pull in plenty of oxygen, it is strengthened and thus functions better. The lungs also have a larger capacity for oxygen.

• **Healthier digestive system** – Drawing in oxygen into the lower abdomen massages the internal organs in the digestive system like the stomach and intestines. A massaged stomach and intestines mean foods move smoothly, lessening the chances of having constipation. Additionally, since deep breathing helps you remain calm even in the face of stressful situations, it can prevent an upset stomach.

• **Improved fitness of the heart** – Pumping blood throughout the body 24/7 is no mean feat. The heart does not fail its function, unless you damage it or if you were born with a congenital heart defect. Other than that, keeping your heart healthy is within your power. Practicing deep breathing aids in keeping the heart healthy by utilizing enough oxygen in circulation.

• **Calmer nervous system** – An abundant supply of oxygen calms the mind and helps you think more clearly.

• **More flexible muscles** – Tension in the muscles that contribute to pain and soreness can be relieved if you are comfortable. A way to relax is to breathe deeply.

• **Increased brainpower** – Taking in much oxygen through deep breathing means that more oxygen goes to the brain and fuels mental processes. The result: better concentration, well thought out decisions, and higher productivity and learning.

• **Emotional relief** – A relaxed body brings out emotional balance and less stress. A relaxed body allows the release of endorphins that facilitate good sleeping habits and lesser feeling of pain.

• **Improved relationships** – Who wouldn't want to have happy and meaningful relationships – whether it be with your spouse, your kids, your siblings, your friends or your co-workers? Deep breathing lets you feel good about yourself and others. When you feel good about yourself and others, you are only minutely bothered, if ever, by the shortcomings of others. You accept others for who they are, with their limitations and strengths. When it comes to your significant other, sexual enjoyment can be expected.

• **More depth** – When you are connected with the things around you as you breathe deeply, your ability to meditate also deepens. Moreover, your depth spills over to your work or some other aspect of your life and shows in your enhanced creativity and intuition.

So when you hear someone say they are going to take a breather, that means they are going to rest or relax. For a real breather where you are not subjected to air pollution, the best quality of air can be found in rural areas with lots of vegetation. Places where there are no smokestacks or vehicles that burn off fossil fuels have more breathable air. Add to that the presence of vegetation, like forests or even prairies; plants give off oxygen as a by-product of photosynthesis. Practicing deep breathing can stimulate your mornings by boosting your energy and fueling your body as you do your tasks. Deep breathing also exercises your lungs and diaphragm.

Given that proper deep breathing has benefits, it is likewise important to know what or which level of air pressure can be beneficial for deep breathing. Air pressure refers to the weight of the air pressing down on the water, the Earth and the air beneath it. You can breathe freely at sea level. When you ascend an elevated region such as a mountain, the air pressure decreases and there is more stress on the lungs. That is why you breathe faster to take in more oxygen.

CHAPTER FIFTEEN:

FIRE IS MOTIVATION

In the physical realm, the sun is considered a source of nourishment because it radiates energy that is used by plants for their own growth. For humans, the light it gives off becomes a source of energy for the skin to make vitamin D that helps absorb calcium. The sun also gives off heat that warms the earth and makes life possible. If not for the warmth of the sun, planet earth would freeze much like Pluto, Neptune or Uranus. No plant, animal or human life could thrive, much less survive on a cold and freezing planet.

Just like the heat and warmth received by the earth from the sun, the human body burns the fuel received from the food eaten. This fuel is converted to energy to power the body's multiple processes, such as digestion, respiration, circulation and movements, among others. The primary source of energy for the body are carbohydrate rich foods like potatoes, bread, cakes, pastries, candies and sugary drinks like powdered fruit juices and soda. If you are on a diet with limited intake of carbohydrates, your body uses fat – specifically, the carbon content of fat. Fat is just a back-up to carbohydrate combustion because fat is less efficiently burned than carbohydrates.

Those who are starving or undernourished in the hopes of losing weight burn protein when there are no more carbohydrate or fat reserves. The amino acids in proteins are transformed into glycogen, which is a form of carbohydrate, to fuel the body. In this manner, you can say that combustion takes place in the body much like gasoline is burned to drive a car. Therefore, fire in whatever appearance, is the mechanism that converts fuel to energy. So what, essentially, is fire? What are its benefits and uses?

More than converting fuel to energy and providing warmth and heat to living things, fire also cleans. In the forest where trees compete with underbrush, a small or controlled fire can remove the underbrush and expose the earth to nourishment by the sun. More nutrients are also absorbed by the trees rather than the underbrush, resulting to better health for the trees. Better health for the trees equates to more food for the birds and other animals. Birds and animals, then, prefer to live in areas where there is abundant food. Places where biodiversity is high can be converted into parks where people can be close to nature.

For people who live near water bodies such as rivers and lakes, fire can be used as a torch during night fishing. For urbanites, fire can be used to convert energy sources like coal and natural gas into electricity that powers most appliances and gadgets. Fire is also used for cooking, for the hearth, barbecue or outdoor picnics, preserving meat and their hides through smoking, removing creases through steam, healing, cauterizing or killing diseases and enjoying tobacco. For artisans and engineers, fire is used for smelting, bending wood through steam, molding glass and making tools. Likewise, fire is an essential component of rituals and ceremonies, including the Olympics.

For campers, having a fire completes the essence of camping. It is the source of light and heat and the means to survive. However, irresponsible use of the resources can leave a negative impact. An example is having a fire on organic soil. This practice kills life on the soil. An alternative is to use mound fires by looking for sand, gravel or mineral soil on which to start a fire. If you are camping on the beach, it is much easier. You can also use fire pans if you have any. If there is an existing fire ring, use it.

Add little bits of wood fuel at a time so you do not create large fires and it takes a little time to burn out when you leave. Do not use branches that are still on trees, even if they are already dead. Use fallen twigs. Leave large wood or logs to decompose; they add nutrients to the soil. When communing with nature, always remember to leave nothing behind – except your footprints. In addition to the survival aspects of camping, it gives you time to meditate as well as allows you to face challenges from the moment that you head to the site and return home.

During this time, you may understand that, ultimately, you hold the power to change your life. The Spartan environment that surrounds you while camping can expose the hidden opportunities that lie around whatever situation you are in when you are in the comfort of your home. Being close to home or living in the city can give you a feeling of ease knowing that gadgets, appliances and what have you are within reach. Being equipped only with the basics lets your creative juices flow and helps you prioritize those that are important to you.

The challenges that you face when camping give you the courage and the will to forge ahead with what you plan to do, knowing that what matters most is the journey, not the destination. The challenge that you may be facing in your daily life may be a new position at work with new responsibilities, grief and emptiness following the loss of a loved one or just an empty nest. While staring at a campfire, you might realize that just like a Phoenix, you will see the change as an opportunity to be reborn.

Being reborn means that you can start a new life but not entirely a different one. It does not mean, though, that you'll have to change everything: new circle of friends, new hobbies or new lifestyle. It just means that you continue doing what you love despite the loss or emptiness. It could mean going the extra mile to accomplish a task or doing things differently but with the goal of achieving or enhancing your productivity. When changes occur in life this gives you the opportunity for constructive and healthy decision to be made.

ENERGIZE – CASE STUDY #2

Gillian McKeith - A nutritionist from Scotland who used to host "You are What You Eat" on a British TV network, Gillian McKeith is one person who believes in the power of fruits and vegetables to boost energy naturally. The show was a dieting program that featured people who lost weight by eating certain kinds of food. McKeith advocates a diet composed mainly of fruits and vegetables coupled with regular exercise. She also advises avoiding sugar and fat, caffeine, high-calorie foods and food that's primarily made of white flour.

Wikipedia. (2014, March 23). Gillian McKeith. Retrieved March 27, 2014, from Wikipedia.org: http://en.wikipedia.org/wiki/Gillian_McKeith

PART V:
"AROUND A FIFTH ONE. A FIFTH… ELEMENT."

"Around A Fifth One. A Fifth… Element."
— Professor Pacoli from the movie The Fifth Element (1997)

"Time is of no importance. Only life is important."
— Father Vito Cornelius

CHAPTER SIXTEEN:

MOVIE SYNOPSIS: THE FIFTH ELEMENT

The movie, "The Fifth Element" is a sci-fi thriller that takes place in the 23rd century. It starts with a scene that happens in 1914. The protectors of the stones that symbolize the four elements as well as a fifth element in the form of a sarcophagus remove the symbols from planet earth since it has been deemed unsafe. Three hundred years later, the fifth element returns to earth but is ambushed by aliens. What remains of the fifth element is a hand that became the basis for giving it rebirth in human body.

The fifth element was tasked to protect the earth in unity with the four stone symbols from the Great Evil. The battle for possession of the stones takes place in a cruise liner, in space. The stones were kept inside the body of an opera singer who dies during the battle. Finally, the stones were retrieved by a human who was guided by a priest and told to proceed directly to the ancient Egyptian temple. Four stone symbols had to be specifically positioned and opened to work in union with the fifth element to stop the Great Evil in the form of a burning spherical mass just like a star.

After figuring out a way to open the stones, the fifth element combines their powers and releases the Divine Light that could stop the Great Evil that was heading toward earth. The Great Evil was stopped just in time and the earth was spared from annihilation.

When the stones were opened and activated, the result was a key formed in the shape of a triangular prism in different colors. The key for wind was yellow, green for earth, blue for water and red for fire. In the movie, the keys had to work together much as in real life for the sustenance of life. Air or wind is needed by life to breathe; the earth produces the food that we eat and water cleanses and nourishes our bodies, as well. Fire is also used to clean and nourish the earth, in order for it to produce healthful food.

The fifth element combines and magnifies the power of the four elements so that it produces a much stronger power. It is a manifestation of the concept that the whole is larger than its parts. In your life, you can also find this unity, thus, resulting to harmony and balance in your lifestyle. Finding peace is not rocket science. Neither is it unachievable. You just have to acknowledge your strengths and limitations. Work with your strengths to achieve higher productivity. Make use of limitations as learning experiences. Knowing your limitations helps you pick out situations or circumstances which will bring out the best in you and those which you can let pass or delegate to someone else.

If you have an idea but you are not good at articulating it, you can still echo out your idea by presenting it in a way that capitalizes on what you can do: as presenting it graphically through a graphic display or infographic or artistically through a play or performance. You may have it supplemented with a good speech from a charismatic speaker. In a way, the movie "The Fifth Element" shows us that we can thrive wherever we are planted. A cab driver in the movie was a former decorated military officer. Just because you no longer work for an institution, like the military, doesn't mean you cannot or you will no longer use the skills you learned previously.

The movie also shows that a higher power can be achieved even with its smaller parts. Alone or singly, each stone cannot function. But with others, it can even save the world.

I first mentioned the concept of aether in the section on the four classical elements. I referred to it as the vastness beyond the terrestrial sphere while the earth, water, air and fire referred to a person's power, intuition, intellect and courage, respectively. In person, achieving balance and harmony means tempering strength with intuition and courage with intellect. That is to say that you can be strong and courageous, but it must be based on your intuition and intellect. You do not just fight for something based on your emotions or what others think. You, yourself have to discern the consequences of your own actions and how it could affect others.

In effect, you direct your own life. You have the power to change it. You are the master of your own ship. You navigate your own course. You are responsible for what you become.

You are the fifth element. Control your space, control your elements. You determine how you use the knowledge of the remaining four elements. You represent a void where all four elements are necessary for vitality. As in the movie Fifth Element, love is the fifth element. Love is the presence of harmony and balance. Love the Art of Living. Embrace the peace. The fifth element is created from the balance and harmony of earth, water, air, and fire; the basic four elements.

CHAPTER SEVENTEEN:

MERIDIANS

When you learn to draw, it is a good way to practice using grid lines so you tackle or work through the entire picture bit by bit. The grid lines are there as guides. Just like when looking at a chart or map, there are meridians. You study a part of the entire chart or map, a space at a time. When you speak of meridians within the body, those are the paths "through which the life-energy known as 'qi' flows," as defined by Wikipedia.[1] So you can say that those are guides upon which pressure or healing is applied.

In utilizing and benefiting from the meridians in our body, we will also encounter chakras, which are "spiritual energy centers located in our spiritual bodies that channel Universal Life force Energy in and out of our spiritual and physical selves," as explained by the website reikirays.com.[2] Therefore, chakras emit life force energy that is transmitted to other points or chakras in the body through meridians. Imagine a map where there is a line of longitude. This imaginary line of longitude is at a right angle to the equator and passes through the north and south poles. In the same way, the body also has meridian lines.

These meridian lines are paired together and total 12 in all. They are also considered as prime meridians since they are the main energy paths in Chinese medicine. Its similarity to the prime meridian in geography is that it marks the origin of the measurement. So a prime meridian is often designated at zero degrees longitude. Six of the meridian lines in the body correspond to the yin while the other six correspond to the yang. Yin and yang are important concepts when working with your life force energy because they are two opposite ideas which must be held in balance so that your overall health is also in balance.

A simple analogy would be that of the line of longitude that passes through the north and south poles; meridian lines go north or south or yin and yang. So a meridian arc, which is the distance between two points within a longitude, refers to the pairing of meridians. Since the pressure point in the hand that refers to the lung is paired with that of the large intestine meridian, a meridian arc exists between the lung and the large intestine. The 12 body meridians are triple warmer, gall bladder, pericardium, liver, kidney, lung, bladder, large intestine, small intestine, stomach, heart and spleen meridians.

The body meridians govern a particular organ's function and their paths which could be blocked if you experience pain or stress in a specific spot of your body. If you feel a headache or earache, then you probably have a blocked triple warmer meridian. Chakras, on the other hand, are energy centers and are believed to be mapped mainly in the midline of your body from the crown of the head to the base of the spine. Let me reiterate that there are 12 energy channels within the body and they form the basis for healing and balance.

Notice that the meridians refer to internal organs yet can be manipulated on certain points in the hands and feet. That is because the meridians make a connection from the outer part of the body toward the internal organs. Chinese meridians also connect to Chinese chakras to enable the transmission of energy from one chakra to another; there are three Chinese chakras – upper, middle and lower dantians. Aside from applying pressure to certain points on the body, particularly the limbs, energy can be allowed to flow by adopting yoga positions that activate yoga meridians.

Reiki also makes use of these meridians or pathways. Through hand positions that are placed on a particular body part which is suffering pain or disease, the life force energy is manipulated to dissolve the blockage, thereby easing the flow of energy. Shiatsu massage also utilizes the presence of the life force energy or qi within the body. Through manual manipulations, like pressing, kneading and tapping, the life force energy is allowed to flow unhindered or unconstricted. In this case, meridians are called vital points and are accessed by a shiatsu practitioner so that energy balance can be restored.

In reflexology, the concept of energy flowing in and out of the body is recognized. Energy that flows in and out of the body can be accessed and activated or stimulated through reflexology meridians. Reflexology meridians are found in the hands, feet and face. Applying certain points to access these meridians can energize and stimulate a specific organ and make it function more efficiently.

Meanwhile, acupressure follows the location and connections of Chinese meridians. So when pain or weakness is felt in a muscle group, it is only a manifestation of an underlying organ, its function or its meridian that is distressed. By distressed, it means that the meridian that is responsible for transporting its energy is congested or irritated. Life force energy is allowed to flow freely by applying pressure on specific points.

When we understand a map, we know how to get from one point

to the other. It guides us on a course to take to reach a destination. Just like geographical maps, the body's meridians guide us as to the flow of human energy. The body's meridians help us to be aware of where our strengths lie and which parts need stimulation to direct the flow of energy so it becomes energized. Awareness of the self guides us to pursue activities that are worthwhile rather than mundane. We become proactive rather than reactive. And we love ourselves for it because we know we have a purpose.

---

[1] Wikipedia. (2014, February 28). Meridian (Chinese Medicine). Retrieved March 4, 2014, from Wikipedia.org: http://en.wikipedia.org/wiki/Meridian_%28Chinese_medicine%29

[2] Reiki Rays. (2012, October 24). How the Meridians and Chakras Work Together? Retrieved March 24, 2014, from reikirays.com: http://reikirays.com/185/how-the-meridians-and-chakras-work-together/

THE *60 SECOND*
CHALLENGE

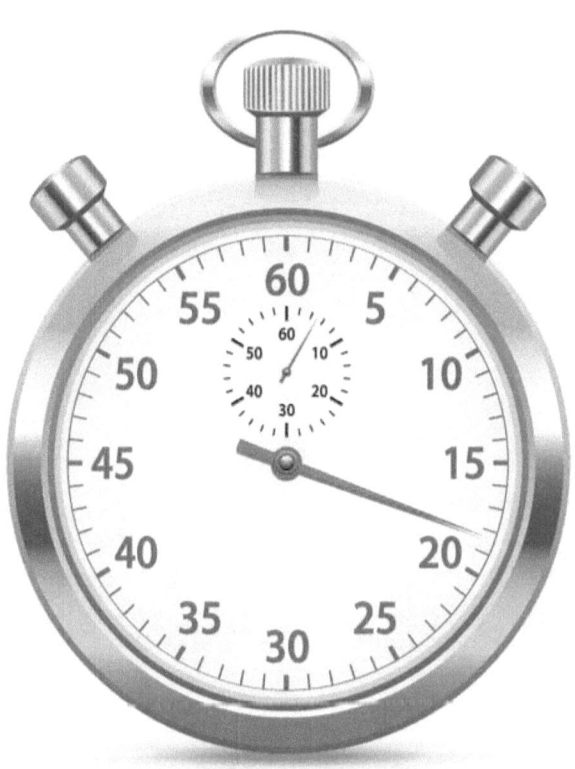

THE QUIZ
Quick Review

1. Name five elements discussed in this book.
2. Name four steps to a relaxation routine.
3. How can I boost my energy, right now?
4. What are two ways to trigger my energy?

It is OK if you did not complete this task in *60 seconds*.

STEP-RELAX-BREATHE *&GO* have a productive day.

ENERGIZE – CASE STUDY #3

Dr. Mehmet Cengiz Oz – Dr. Oz as he is commonly known is the face you see on "The Dr. Oz Show." He is a cardiovascular surgeon and teaches at Columbia University. He recognizes the presence of energy in the body and as a cardiovascular surgeon, allows Reiki healing during heart transplant operations and open heart surgeries.

Desy, P. I. (n.d.). Doctor Mehmet Oz. Retrieved March 27, 2014, from healing.about.com: http://healing.about.com/od/famoushealers/p/mehmet-oz.htm

CHAPTER EIGHTEEN:

THE ENERGIZE CASE STUDIES

You can see that other people have resorted to alternative medicine to deal with certain conditions. The philosophies that guide alternative medicine are incorporated into their lifestyles. There are also people who have adopted practices in alternative medicine even though they are not experiencing debilitating conditions. Some may not have undergone bad experiences but saw someone, perhaps a loved one suffer from devastating experiences.

Even in everyday instances, changing your lifestyle to follow the precepts of alternative medicine can be rewarding. Doing regular exercise can boost your energy, strengthen your muscles and immune system and decrease your risk of having a heart attack or stroke. Increasing your nutrient intake through energy juicing can also beef up your health. Meditation or prayer is practiced to add dimension for a well-balanced life. Massages have become important methods to relieve stress and induce relaxation. The presence of life force energy within the body is taken advantage of through healing techniques as Reiki or acupuncture.

As of now, methods used in alternative medicine have been considered in treating health conditions. For example, using acupuncture in treating asthma is used instead of just supplementing them to orthodox, allopathic therapies. Yoga has also been recommended in treating chronic back pain.

You have many choices in dealing with physical, as well as mental and emotional health problems. You can choose the oft-taken path of conventional medicine which most likely deals with your health problem only physically. Or you can choose alternative medicine that addresses your mental and emotional states on top of your physical wellbeing. Choosing alternative medicine entails following the natural way of healing. One way to achieve the natural way of healing is to recognize the presence of energy centers or chakras and energy pathways or meridians. Manipulating or stimulating such centers and pathways can loosen energy congestion somewhere in your body.

Stimulating these centers and pathways also need changes in lifestyle which include regular exercise, a healthy diet, meditation, practicing healthy breathing techniques, taking in the sun for your supply of vitamin D and good sleeping habits. These things may take some time of getting used to, but the benefits may be worth your while. Remember: no pain, no gain.

BONUS ELEMENTS

CHAPTER NINETEEN:

COFFEE: MAINTAINING AND BOOSTING YOUR ENERGY LEVELS

There are lots of mixed perceptions regarding coffee and its main ingredient – caffeine. Nevertheless, many people cannot get through the day without their caffeine fix. Most of them take it in the afternoon, when they need an energy boosting stimulant. The caffeine in coffee acts as a stimulant and doesn't require a prescription. It only takes 10 minutes from the intake of caffeine to experience its effects: energy levels are increased, performance is enhanced and productivity rises. Performance is enhanced because the caffeine in coffee blocks adenosine – which encourages sleep and suppresses arousal – while increasing substances in the brain that promote general cognitive function, memory and mood.

Coffee is also a fat burner. Again, the caffeine content of coffee not only boosts energy levels but your metabolic rate, as well. Caffeine is a natural substance that helps burn fat. That is why it is usually found in fat-burning supplements. Since it can only burn so much, it should be coupled with regular exercise to see amazing results. Drinking coffee 30 minutes before regular exercise helps the body raise adrenaline levels so that the body can keep up even with strenuous activities. Fatty acids that have been stored will be used as fuel for such activities.

Not only is coffee a stimulant, but it is also a nutritious drink. Coffee beans themselves contain B-complex vitamins and minerals which find their way into the roasted and ground beverage that many people enjoy. There are also many ways of enjoying it. Aside from drinking it in its classic black instant state, it can be enjoyed as an Espresso, Café Americano, Café au lait or Latte. Milk, cream, and tea are flavored with sugar, honey or cinnamon. It is even a garnishing or ingredient in various desserts as an affogato, ice cream or cakes.

Interestingly, coffee has been shown to reduce the risk of several diseases, including cancers of the lungs, prostate, breast, colon, stomach, pancreas or uterus. Due to the presence of antioxidants in coffee. These natural substances prevent or delay cell damage. Likewise, coffee lowers the likelihood of getting heart disease or stroke. A healthy heart and healthy blood pressure are attained by regularly drinking coffee and making sure the caffeine in it gets metabolized. Metabolizing caffeine can be achieved when one engages in physical activity rather than be a couch potato. Simple brisk walking or jogging can already do this.

Aside from cancers and heart disease, coffee has been associated with a lower risk of getting type II diabetes. Type II diabetes is a growing health concern and afflicts even children. This condition raises blood sugar levels and makes its sufferers insulin resistant. The risk of getting type II diabetes through regular intake of coffee may be averted because of its caffeine content which burns fat. Obese people are more likely to get this disease so that helping their bodies burn fat also lowers their risk. However, drinking coffee is not enough. They should also have a healthy diet and maintain a healthy blood sugar level.

Though coffee is shown to be beneficial, they must be taken in properly. Having it early in the morning without eating food first stimulates the body to make hydrochloric acid which can irritate an empty stomach. Otherwise, undigested meals can lead to bloating, irritable bowel syndrome or gas. Irritation of the gut can also pave the way for a bacterium – responsible for ulcers – to take hold. If your body is sensitive to this beverage, you make experience elimination problems like diarrhea or constipation, cramps and abdominal spasms.

Another side effect to drinking coffee is heartburn. Since the muscles of the throat have a tendency to relax after drinking coffee or any caffeinated beverage, the food that you have eaten may come back up and cause heartburn. Heartburn is especially true for pregnant women. What you can do – whether pregnant or not – is not to lie down after eating. Help your digestive system do its work by sitting-up to make sure that food is directed downward. On the other hand, drinking coffee may promote the quick transport of food from the stomach and intestines into the anus for elimination. Nutrients may not be absorbed by the body from the food that you eat. So if you have to drink coffee, do it in the afternoon when you have finished lunch.

Drinking coffee in the evening should not be done too late so that it does not interfere with your sleep cycle. Remember that coffee blocks adenosine to make you alert. Drinking coffee at least six hours before bedtime is okay since coffee and its effects last for only about three hours and can get eliminated from the body through urine after that.

As alcoholic beverages, too many cups of coffee can free up stress hormones like epinephrine, norepinephrine and cortisol so that there is a feeling of tension rather than relaxation. Similarly, it can interfere with your digestion and bring on more health problems. So instead of drinking too much coffee when you feel overwhelmed by work or personal anxieties, take time for meditation to regain your balance and attain harmony for a good health. Enjoying a cup of coffee twice a day may be good for your health and improve the quality of life. As with all things, take it in moderation.

Black Coffee, No Sugar, No Cream

From the immortal words of Dwight Errington Myers, better known as Heavy D, "Black coffee, no sugar, no cream" are lyrics from his 1994 smash hit, "Black Coffee." If you do choose to have coffee think about reducing the amount of sweetener, cream, and intake of refined sugars. Caffeine is not the only way you can boost your energy in the morning.

CHAPTER TWENTY:

OH! AND THERE ARE SIDE EFFECTS

As your body benefits from the effects of naturally boosting your energy, there are also some side effects to consider. Here are seven side effects you are sure to notice.

1. The most obvious side effect is clear skin. You will notice a change but the others will notice it more than you. Your standards trump status quo when it comes to your skin. Other people will feel compelled to comment on your radiant skin.

2. Your nails will not only grow faster but grow stronger

3. The same goes for your hair. Your hair will not only

grow faster but grow stronger, thicker, and shinier

4.   The second most obvious is the boost in energy will become addictive. The same way you notice if you skipped the premium gas for the regular unleaded. As you hit the gas your vehicle responses different.

5.   As you respect your temple; you adversely begin to open the world to that body of respect

6.   I have mentioned all this talk about deep breathing and haven't told you that even your breath smells fresher. Good bye to morning breath. Think about it if you are ingesting natural nutrients your body will seldom reject it unless you have a medical reaction to some nutrients. Morning breath is the body rejecting unnatural elements. I notice more morning breath after drinking a refreshment with high fructose corn syrup. Your body was not created to digest this artificial sweetener

7.   Muscle regeneration. If you increase your physical activities, including weight lifting, your muscles will have enough fuel and nutrients to regenerate itself. You will feel less pain as your sore muscles grow.

CHAPTER TWENTY-ONE

THE ENERGY CHECKLIST

11 THINGS TO KNOW ABOUT NATURAL ENERGY BOOSTERS

As we get older and take on more responsibilities, we can start to feel run down. When we do not keep our life in balance and our health at the top of our priority list, it can affect our energy levels not to mention our overall health. Here are 11 things you need to know about naturally boosting your energy from alternative medicine to self-healing methods. Just being mindful of your energy is a start. From 60-second energy boosts to a running a marathon tap into your energy source.

1. **Our diets greatly affect our energy levels**. Food is fuel after all. Those who don't skip breakfast have been shown to be in a better mood and have more energy throughout the day. The journal Nutritional Health published studies that determined those that missed any meal during the day felt more fatigued by the end of the day. Eating a balanced diet is crucial to health and wellbeing. When you are getting enough vitamins and minerals your body can function optimally. One very essential mineral is Magnesium, which is needed for over 300 biochemical reactions in the body including the breakdown of glucose into energy.

2. **Eating too many foods containing refined sugar can affect your blood sugar and, therefore, your energy levels, as well**. Sugars create a burst of energy than a rapid drop in blood sugar as well as energy levels. Cutting out or reducing processed foods will give the body real foods as fuel, and the body was built to run on real food. The reduction or elimination of processed foods will help the body to operate optimally, without the distractions of toxins or extra work to digest, etc.

3. **Not drinking enough water affects energy levels**. Water makes up 50-60 percent of the human body and no other substance is as widely involved in all the processes and makeup of our bodies. That makes it the most important nutrient we can ingest. We can go weeks without food but without water we only last several days. We feel thirsty when the water in our body is reduced by only 1 percent! When it is reduced by 5 percent we become hot and tired because muscle strength and endurance declines significantly. Sometimes when we are even slightly dehydrated we can feel tired and lethargic according to nutritionist Keith Ayoob, EdD, RD. What an easy fix a glass of water can provide! Water keeps our cells running smoothly and our energy levels up.

4.   Reduce and manage your stress. Stress is a big energy killer. Stress and anxiety drains a good amount of our energy – even if you've spent the day in bed. Low, chronic levels of stress slowly and surely chip away at energy levels. Identify what kind of activities are most relaxing for you and engage, even if it is just talking on the phone, because it will reduce your tension and increase your energy. EFT (Emotional Freedom Technique) is a priceless (yet completely free!) tool for not only reducing stress, but overcoming major and minor issues that keep coming up and draining your energy. EFT also physically taps the thymus that triggers the production of T-cells and boosts energy.

5.   Learn some basic acupressure for more energy and better health. To understand acupressure, one needs to understand meridians. These are pathways that connect certain "points" on the body to each other and to the internal organs. Think of how blood vessels carry the life giving blood that physically nourishes the body. Meridians are similar but instead they circulate electrical power. Western medicine calls this our nervous system, but it is so much more than that. Imbalances developed in this energy flows causing some of the "points" to become congested or irritated. This results in weakness and sometimes pain in the surrounding area, specifically the muscles. When we stimulate these "points" via acupressure (or acupuncture) we help to normalize the imbalance, even if it is something simple like low energy or fatigue.

6.   Practice reflexology for a boost in energy levels. Reflexology might be considered a sister to acupressure. There are a couple theories behind reflexology but the underlying theme is that there are areas on the feet and hands ("reflex" areas) that correspond to specific parts of the body, including organs, glands, etc. For example, the liver, pancreas and kidney are in the arch of the foot and the head is reflected in the tips of the toes. This practice has been around since Ancient

Egyptian times. Practitioners apply pressure to certain reflex areas to promote health in the corresponding organ/gland via the body's natural energy pathways. Reflexology uses the body's own power to heal itself. A couple reflexology massages can help increase energy. Often fatigue comes when blood sugar levels are low. The pancreas is involved with blood sugar regulation so working the "pancreas reflex" a few times a day can help. Working the adrenal reflex will help adrenaline levels and, therefore, help boost energy.

7.   **Get your daily dose of sunshine**. The skin uses the energy from sunlight to produce the hormone, vitamin D, which is what boosts energy levels. The active form of vitamin D is now thought to regulate at least one thousand different genes that govern almost every tissue in the body. Bones do not form properly without sufficient vitamin D. When this happens in children they develop a disease called Rickets that is characterized by slow growth and skeletal deformities as the hallmark bowed legs. While the sun is best known for boosting production of vitamin D, it is responsible for other important effects. For example, UVR from the sun raises levels of natural opiates called endorphins in our blood. Sun exposure will cause an overall increase in feelings of well-being and, therefore, an increased sense of energy. Soaking up sunshine for 15-20 minutes energizes the body and elevates mood.

8.   **Increasing physical activity, even something as simple as going for a walk, increases energy levels**. Dr. Robert Thayer, at California State University, discovered that a brisk 10-minute walk increased energy in the test subjects. They also felt the effects for up to two hours. The increase in energy is good news since walking is easy to do and can be done anywhere! Regular exercise, even walking, also raises those feel-good endorphins.

9.   **Incorporate active stretching into your daily life**. Stretching provides numerous benefits to the body including

increased energy levels, greater blood circulation in certain parts of the body and relief from stress. Improved circulation allows an increase of blood flow to the muscles and joints. In turn, this brings more nutrients to our cells while also removing waste byproducts and toxins. Proper stretching helps to relax tense muscles. Relief from tension brings on an overall feeling of well-being and increased energy.

10.   When your body gets enough sleep, your brain can commit things to memory easier. Sleep also helps to keep your metabolism and hormone levels within the ideal range as well boosts overall health, immunity and energy. Even though sleep is known to prevent aging by giving the body time to repair damage and rejuvenate, it is, unfortunately, an incredibly underutilized anti-aging tool.

11.   The benefits of deep breathing might be a little surprising at first, considering how easily one can learn this exercise. Deep breathing releases endorphins throughout the body. The oxygen we inhale provide energy removing toxins from our organs that result in better blood flow. Other benefits of deep breathing include a reduction in stress and blood pressure, relief of general body aches and better sleep. All these benefits result in an overall increase, in energy levels. When we very simply breathe deeply we are helping our overall health.

The *60 Second* Boost

Just being mindful of your energy is a start.

www.60secondboost.com.

Chapter Twenty-Two:

The Double **P.L.A.Y.Y.** Approach

PLAN to feel energized.

Best time to plan is in the mornings when your day begins.

LISTEN to your changing body.

As your body develops, start to pay attention to what foods your body craves. Moderation is the key to controlling your food binge.

ADAPT the fundamentals.

Adapt the elegant knowledge of this book to every moment of your life.

YIN and YANG

Balance is the key. Breathe in, breathe out. Be mindful.

YELLOW SUN

Get your daily dose of sunshine. Let the sun be your catalyst.

CHAPTER TWENTY-THREE:

MORE CASE STUDIES

Energy boosting techniques are advocated and taught by some people and multiple organizations. There are well-known people who recognize the efficacy of natural energy boosting as well as the existence of energy within the body. Here are some additional case studies for review:

Dr. Andrew Weil

Dr. Andrew Weil – Dr. Andrew Weil is known to advocate the

marriage of Western medicine and alternative therapies. He obtained his medical degree from Harvard University and established the Arizona Center for Integrative Medicine based in the University of Arizona. He specifically encourages integrating the intake of omega-3 fatty acids, a healthy dose of vitamin D and some meditation with those of doctors' prescriptions.

Janet Mentgen

Janet Mentgen – Healing Touch International Inc. is an organization founded by nurse, Janet Mentgen. The organization has been acknowledged by the American Holistic Nurses Association and the Canadian Holistic Nurses Association. It offers instruction and training on energy-based therapy and certifies learners after level three of its training program. Trainees can become instructors after they have completed level five of the program.

Dr. Frank Lipman

Dr. Frank Lipman – Dr. Frank Lipman believes in benefitting from the positive attributes of both western medicine and eastern healing philosophies. To complement his medical training as an internist, Dr. Lipman has studied acupuncture, Chinese medicine, nutrition, meditation and yoga and came up with a wellness center to help people get back their energy and passion for life.

Randomized Controlled Trials

A review of randomized controlled trials using acupressure to treat symptoms experienced during pregnancy and chemotherapy – like vomiting and nausea – yielded 70% success in 23 such trials. Other conditions involving the use of acupressure to treat pain during labor, dysmenorrhea and after trauma resulted to a 90% success rate.

Severe Psoriasis

A man with severe psoriasis due to his arthritis tried reflexology. He had difficulty in walking due to lesions in his legs and his sleep was often disturbed by the itching and burning brought about by the sores. Over the course of his sessions, it was found out that the reflex points in his feet indicated problems in his neck, lymphatic system, kidney, large intestine, his gut and his lower back. His reflexology sessions were also supplemented with a minor change in diet by increasing water intake and cutting back on caffeine. After eight reflexology sessions, he noticed an improvement in his sleep patterns and felt less pain in his neck.

Infertility Issues

Women who feel deprived of motherhood because of infertility issues now have hope in the form of Reiki healing. A woman who had polycystic ovary syndrome (PCOS) looked for alternatives to clinical treatment. She discovered Reiki and took four hourly sessions.

During these sessions, the Reiki practitioner would focus the life force energy of a woman on her reproductive system. Aside from being able to conceive just a few months later after the first session, the woman also felt serene and calm. The Reiki session not only addressed her fertility problem but also her feelings of depression.

Pregnancy Massages

Pregnant women can benefit from massages while pregnant. In the case of shiatsu, where pressure applied by the fingers, it can primarily induce relaxation in women. Due to the unique needs of pregnant women, shiatsu practitioners help them find positions that will eventually help them experience labor less painfully. In fact, massages and breathing techniques form part of a Lamaze class. Furthermore, pregnancy massages given after the first trimester improves sleep, lowers anxiety, decreases stress as well as back and leg pain.

EPILOGUE

A FATHER'S LESSON

"He didn't tell me how to live; he lived, and let me watch
him do it."

— Clarence Budington Kelland

A father's love contributes as much, and sometimes even more
than a mother's love to a child's development and the importance of a
father's love should motivate many men to become more involved in
nurturing their children (Society for Personality and Social Psychology,
2012).[1]

For a woman getting pregnant for the first time, it means that her
essence as a woman is completed and defined. For a man being a father
and a dad for the first time, means their transformation self-absorption
to selflessness. Many fathers can attest that upon seeing their child for
the first time, the feeling of wanting to protect and care for that baby is
instinctive and overwhelming. Fatherhood does not only mean loving
your child and supporting him, but also means, especially when the
child is a boy, to be a role model to him and teach him invaluable
lessons that he will use as a shield and weapon in battling life's
hardships.

My father Dr. Jacques M. Polanco, M.D. was an anesthesiologist
who was married to his Queen, Vanote S. Polanco, R.N.. Being a
student of medicine, my father understands that victory loves
preparation and he applied such norm in his life by continually
studying and taking medical exams to further his knowledge and
improve his skills and capabilities. He passed on this value that he had
in life by constantly motivating me to explore the world and experience
life at its best and worst because he knows that by experiencing enough
out in the real world, I would be able to learn important lessons that
will help me in preparing for life's constant battles.

But my father was not only a student of medicine. He was also a student of the arts. My father's artworks were one of the strongest motivators and constant guide that I carry with me. He showed his love for me by being supportive and by encouraging me to do my best in every endeavor I undertook. By allowing me to be independent and learn lessons from my mistakes. These lessons helped me to set uncomfortable goals in life. And consequently taught me to live by example.

Dr. Polanco being a good provider and good structure to lean on in times of troubles completed my circle of life which was started by my mother's unconditional and unfailing love for me. But my father was not only a provider, he was also a friend who listens to me and respects my decisions because he knows that by allowing me to grow as a man on my own will help me be as strong and as compassionate. Dad did not only teach me how to be a better man. He also gave me a part of his life and part of his ingenuity as a person. I always say that I have my mother's heart and understanding, but I am also proud to say that I have my father's creativity and structure.

Often in life, and this is unavoidable, we make decisions that we often regret in the end. My father did indeed criticize some of my decisions, but one thing he did instill is never to be idle. Dad also served as one of my greatest inspirations in life. The way he lived his life inspired me to become like him; if not to be better than him. Dad did not only dictate life lessons. Instead, he lived his life as best as he could and let me watch him do it and it was the best example that any child could get from their father.

My father taught me how to be strong and man-up whenever problems and trials are trying to push me to the ground. His strength came from years of discipline, precision and endurance in the field of medicine; the same control, precision and endurance that made him a successful man in his career; the same control, precisions and endurance that made me the man that I am today. One of his valuable teachings is that victory and success are in the preparation, and that preparation is empowered through determination. My father showed me through his actions to respect people by treating people the way you want to be treated is also the best way that you can earn their respects. Think before you speak.

So are a father's love, lessons and teaching valuable to a child's life? Yes, it is because, without it, the circle of influence and love will never be complete. We must always remember that our identity came from two beings: our mother and our father. Without examples of masculinity and femininity, life will feel less complete, so cherish your father's love. Learn from his lessons and never forget his teachings because all of these coupled with a mother's unconditional life will be the greatest weapon that one can have in surmounting all the challenges of life.

I would like to share two particular quotes that keep me motivated and focused:

"I decided to take control of my life: I would become a warrior-scholar. I made up my mind to turn my body into a weapon… a weapon that would eventually set me free!"

— Rubin "Hurricane" Carter

"I hated every minute of training, but I said, 'Don't quit. Suffer now and live the rest of your life as a champion.'"

— Mohammed Ali

— FATHER TIME —

---

[1] (2012). Society for Personality and Social Psychology. ScienceDaily. Retrieved March 1, 2014 from http://www.sciencedaily.com/releases/2012/06/120612101338.htm.

I Will Fill In The Blank

I can find 60 seconds to increase my energy while waiting
for _____ ?

Conclusion

Knowing now that energy boosting is right within your fingertips, you can already make changes to your lifestyle. They may not be radical so that you are not overwhelmed by the changes and be discouraged if you neglect to do some in a day or two – like exercise. What is important is that you know that you need to change and that you can accommodate what you are able to without being pressured. You also know that stress comes with the package called life, but it does not mean there's nothing you can do about it.

Even with a hectic schedule, you can squeeze in a few moments throughout your day to increase your physical activity or do breathing exercises. A 60-second physical activity may only mean walking the length from your car to your workplace or taking the stairs. It might also mean a few repetitions of diaphragmatic breathing or it might mean consuming an entire glass of carrot juice, sweetened with honey. On the occasion, you might need a sudden boost of energy for that brainstorming meeting so you resort to a cup of coffee with sugar. That is not entirely bad.

Add to that the information that each of us possesses human healing power. It is the power that anyone can harness. Tapping into your own energy requires the knowledge of what areas to stimulate or manipulate so that human energy can flow unhindered. When your human energy is unhindered, you feel the vitality that doesn't make you crash after a few hours. Moreover, manipulating human energy and letting it flow can alleviate any pain you may be feeling. It can also bring on a feeling of relaxation that relieves you of stress or even depression.

Being familiar with your level of energy also benefits your health. You might get tired easily because you may not be eating right. When you do not eat right, your body's systems may not also be functioning at optimal levels. You could have elevated blood sugar or blood pressure levels. This elevation could heighten your risk for diabetes, heart disease or stroke. So, to make sure that you decrease your risk, you eat healthful foods like fresh vegetables and fruits. You also make a habit of making healthy breathing exercises. Since you take the time to breathe deeply, you might as well match it by increasing your physical activity.

Increasing your physical activity may just mean increasing your time or distance when you walk the dog or simply jog. You can also engage in a sport like swimming, running or skiing. Otherwise, you can also spend more bonding time with your family through camping, having picnics or going fishing. Such projects can also present you with challenges that could bring out the best and creative part of you. When you have spent your waking hours in a productive and enjoyable manner, it is time for you to get some good sleep. Sleeping at least eight hours during the night is beneficial to your overall health – and that includes your mental health.

If, during the day, you feel sluggish or sleepy, thirty minutes might be all it takes for you to take a power nap and regain back energy for work in the afternoon. All throughout the day and all throughout your life, be mindful of the things you do or don't do. A healthy diet, regular exercise, deep breathing and good sleeping habits are the vital ingredients for a productive life. But you most likely grew up being nurtured. So the basic pampering you had as a child should continue until old age. It is up to you to nurture yourself as an adult.

As an adult, you have more choices in nurturing your physical self as well as your mental and emotional self. As an adult, you can try acupressure, acupuncture or reflexology. These therapies take care of the tensions and pain you may be feeling because of the responsibilities you have as an adult. The use of pressure points in such therapies helps the practitioner identify which areas stressed or congested and allow them to remove or relieve the stress. Thus, you pamper yourself.

Pampering and nurturing yourself are not limited to these therapies. There are also relaxation methods, such as deep breathing, yoga, meditation and massage. You can also loosen the muscles that have created tension within your body only by stretching. Likewise, you can lessen the chances for stress, depression and anxiety by living in the present and not worrying about what could happen in the future. You need not worry about the future if you know that what you need is all around you. Take a hint from the four elements: earth, water, air and fire.

You can achieve a healthy diet just by taking the produce of the earth in their natural state. The earth yields fruits and vegetables which supply you with the nutrients you need. Take them as they are or as energy juices. Taking them in their processed states, such as preserves or dried form means ingesting a lot more sugar, preservatives and other additives which aren't good for your body. You can wash down the food with pure water or naturally flavored ones. In addition to the food that you eat, nourish your body with needed calcium with the help of vitamin D from the sun. Lastly, inhale an abundant amount oxygen every time you breathe by learning breathing exercises that increase your lung capacity for oxygen.

When you try different energy boosting techniques you must first be familiar with how they can be acquired. Aside from what nature has to offer, be familiar also with where meridians are. Meridians are also natural energy pathways that exist in all of us. Knowledge of meridians will give you an idea as to which part of the body is congested, damaged or weakened. Determining the affected body part tells you how to manipulate an area so that the balance is restored. A balanced life also helps you get more out of life because you are not dragged down by negativity and you accomplish more because of your positive disposition.

Learning the peak hours that are part of learning about human energy and how to boost it enable you to schedule activities based on which body parts are at their peak performance. It entails going with the flow. Notice how you use up less energy when you are swimming with the current rather than against it? Your ability to read illustrations of meridians also helps you regulate your diet and your lifestyle. If, for example, you seem to be anemic or have a poor immune system, you'll know that your kidney needs some help. So you drink a lot more water, include string beans or celery in your diet and keep track of your cholesterol, blood pressure and blood glucose levels.

In summary, familiarizing yourself with the body's meridians teaches you to adopt a lifestyle that keeps you healthy and fit. You make an effort to exercise regularly to keep your blood pressure and blood sugar in check and at the same time, go for foods high in nutritional value. You learn to control your emotions instead of being overwhelmed by them. Controlling emotions help you overcome anxiety. You can do this if you practice yoga and supplement it with deep breathing exercises. In a complicated world... Look to the elegance and simplicity of nature for lasting truths and solutions of a productive lifestyle.

Acknowledgements

Thank you to the Almighty,
Thank you to the Universe,
Thank you mom, Vanote S. Polanco, R.N.,
Thank you dad, Jacques M. Polanco, M.D.,
Thank you Friends and Family,
Thank you Prince Polanco,
and Thank You for thanking the time to read these words.

From The Author

As you read this you are in the present as time passes we radiate out like ripples in a pond. As we radiate we shed years. We all share presence. Age is just for identification amongst others. Experience is the moments we share. Experience, Dream, and Execute Your Choice.

Live life as an art form. Your life, your masterpiece.

THE ART OF LIVING.

Imagine if you can harvest all the energy boosting techniques to start off your mornings. How would your day be? Would you feel more active and focused to be mindfully productive?

Join the conversation on **www.morningmats.com**

Life is a culmination of experiences. Be mindful of your ways. Learn every day. Evolve. Thank you for taking the time to read this book. See you at **www.60secondboost.com** for exclusive access.

Credits

About The Author

JACQUES POLANCO is a mindful entrepreneur, author, adventurer and artist creating in his hometown of New York City and worldwide. He believes that art is a lifestyle, and behind every art form expresses a fundamental science of harmony.

www.jacquespolanco.com